The little book of BIG Os

Brilliant ideas to take you to the limit

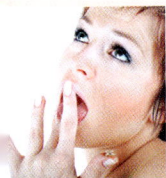

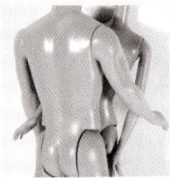

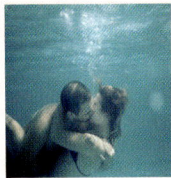

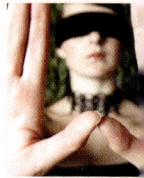

The little book of big Os

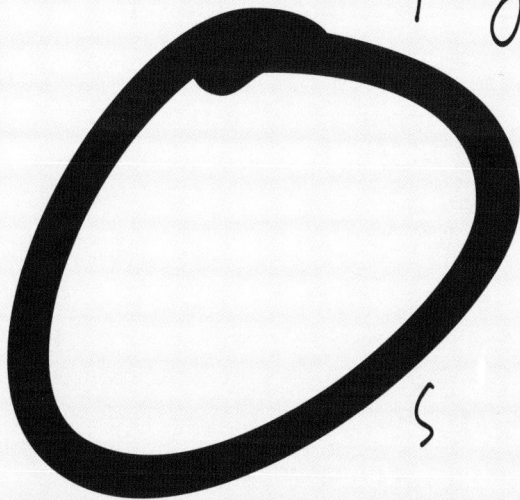

Brilliant ideas to take you to the limit

Marcelle Perks & Elisabeth Wilson

Careful now

Sex can be a risky activity. It's just much more fun if you don't have to worry about a potential unwanted pregnancy or picking up a sexually transmitted infection. So go easy, use plenty of lube and see your doctor in the first instance if you experience problems. Play safe!

Although the contents of this book were checked at the time of going to press, information is constantly changing, especially on the Internet. This means the publisher and author cannot guarantee the contents of any of the websites mentioned in the text.

First published in 2007 by
The Infinite Ideas Company Limited
36 St Giles, Oxford, OX1 3LD, United Kingdom
www.infideas.com

A CIP catalogue record for this book is available from the British Library
ISBN 13: 978-1-904902-92-8
ISBN 10: 1-904902-92-8

Designed and typeset by Baseline Arts Ltd, Oxford
Printed in Singapore

Brilliant ideas

"If sex is such a natural phenomenon, how come there are so many books on how to?"

BETTE MIDLER

Introduction

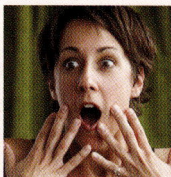

There's no specific audience for this book. You have to be female because it's aimed at women, but there's something for everyone whether you're still a virgin or an experienced seductress. Perhaps you're young, or maybe you're already a great-grandmother; some of you might have to push the boat out to work around your physical disabilities, others will have mental blocks that make their lives difficult. Whatever point we start off from, all of us have our positive points and 'shadow' sides to wrestle with.

The main aim is to help you improve your sex life, and although we can't guarantee you'll have an orgasm (about 10% of women say they *never* climax) there are lots of ideas here that will at least put some fun and interest back into the mix. There are plenty of practical tips and tricks for better techniques to help you along, but they're accompanied by parts devoted to improving your mental outlook. Good sex really is a mixture of biology and psychology.

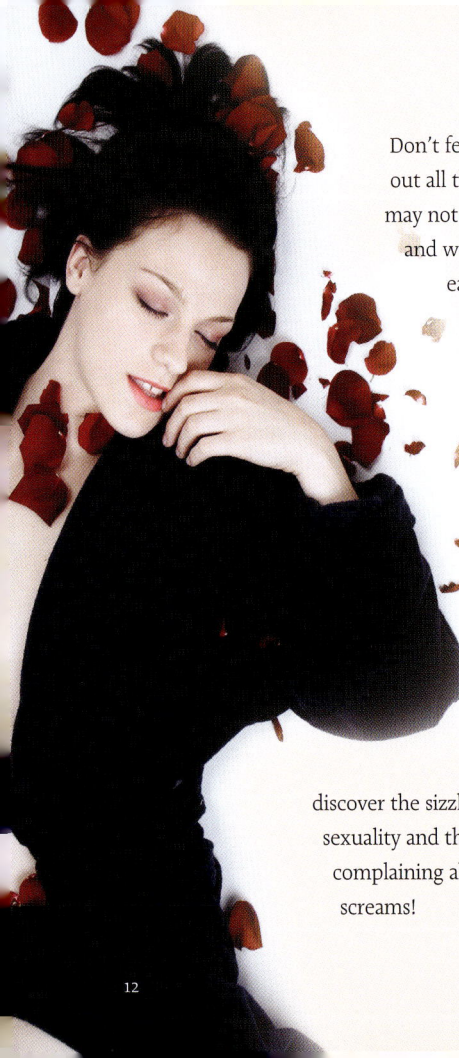

Don't feel that you have to try out all the suggestions. Some may not be appropriate for you and we haven't road-tested each and every one ourselves. There's an honest attempt to present the real deal, warts and all, rather than saccharine secrets for Stepford Wives.

What we've got in common is that we're all looking for 'it'. We hope this book helps you to discover the sizzling side to your sexuality and that the neighbours start complaining about your blissful screams!

1

Sexual thoughts

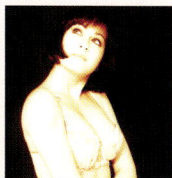

Before we even think physical, we need to probe the most important bit — what's on your mind.

In theory, expressing our sexuality has never been easier. Women now have more opportunities and freedom, a range of contraceptive options, speed dating, online chat sites and amazing sex aids. You'd think we've never had it so good, and yet, according to the Durex 2004 Global Sex Survey, only 35% of women climax every time they have sex. Studies show around 40% of women suffer from sexual dysfunction and about a fifth of us have low levels of libido. Around 10% of women claim they never have orgasms. That means most of us have room for improvement.

Sometimes it's hard to switch off and become sexual. During a sexual encounter anything and everything can get in the way, and women are more likely to be distracted by stray thoughts. To avoid this, practise relaxation and focus exercises. For example, jump into a cold swimming pool and relish the shock you feel in the first few seconds. Later think back to how your body felt and imagine giving over to just this sensation. Take this technique with you to the bedroom and concentrate on good physical sensations. Forget about the holy grail of orgasm. Think of it as a bonus, but that the scenic route, long and meandering, has its plus points too.

Imagine you are your partner telling someone else about what you're like in bed. Highlight your good points, and list any features that are particularly sexy. See how many positive things you can relate about yourself. Often we exaggerate, but the little white lies could later become reality!

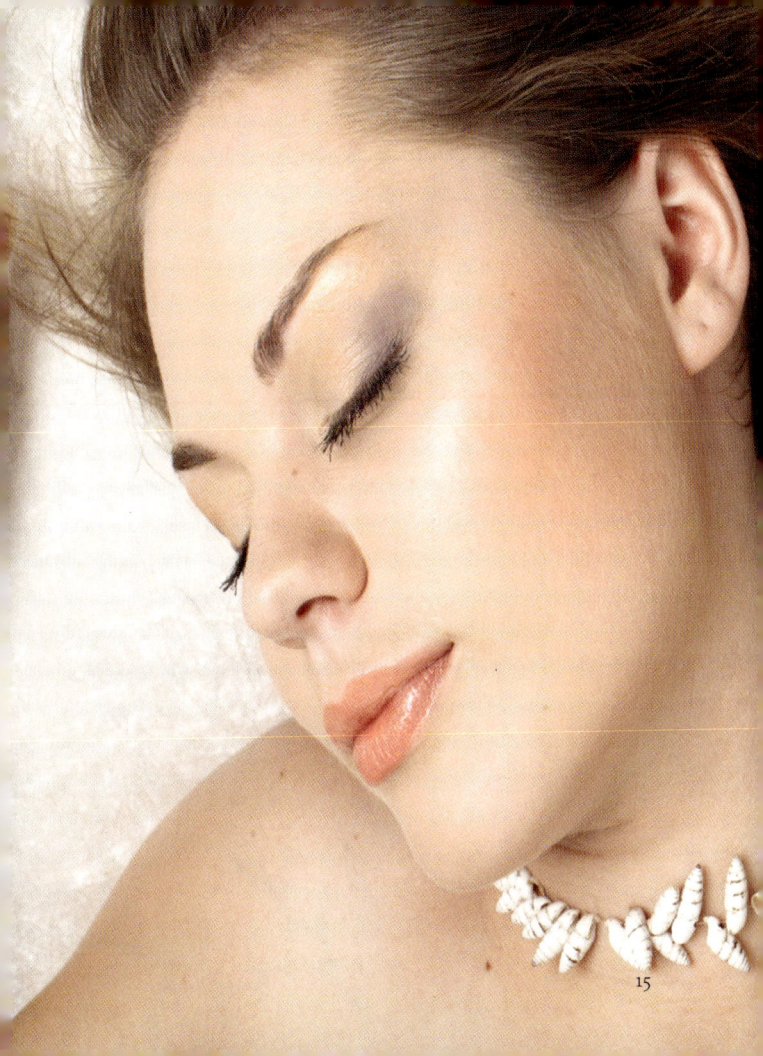

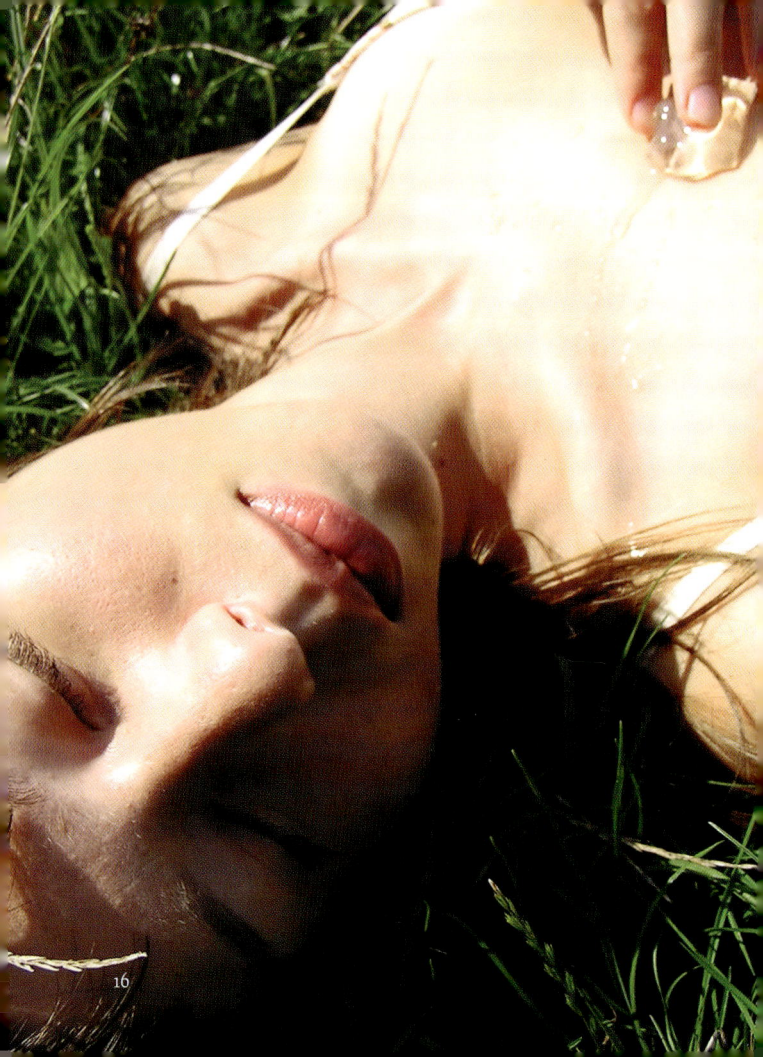

2

Solo player

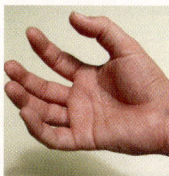

Being able to 'get off' alone means more intense orgasms with someone else.

One of the best ways to maintain your sex drive is to set regular pleasure sessions – with yourself. Some feel a little dirty when they indulge, others frig themselves frantically in front of their partners, but sex researchers estimate that around 80% of women of all ages masturbate, and that means most of us are doing it.

Open your legs wide; the sensation of air should feel pleasant. Wriggle your hips and wait until your labia lips are swollen: this will increase sensitivity and moisture. Dip an exploratory finger just inside your vaginal lips. Use the dribble of moisture on your finger to run your finger around your vaginal lips. You might want to experiment with the perineum – the skin between the vagina and the anus. Try circles, figures of eight, and even tapping motions with your hand. What feels good? You should be nice and moist. Perhaps your clitoris is already retracting from its little hood of skin.

Now is a good time to explore your clitoris. Feel for the clitoris and see which way and what type of strokes feel good. If it doesn't feel sensitive, try using your other hand to pull your skin away from the clitoris. At the same time, look for a second erogenous zone to maximise your pleasure. This could be a finger or two in the vagina, massaging your outer lips, or some form of anal stimulation. You might want to use a vibrator, anal butt plug or some other toy to help you along.

3

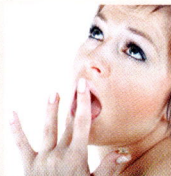

Sticky fingers

Understand your body and tune into your natural cycle.

There are several ways to chart your fertility signs: vaginal mucus, waking temperature and the position of the cervix. The easiest sign to spot is vaginal mucus which changes as you progress through your cycle. After your period, mucus is dry or non-existent. In the second week, as ovulation approaches, it becomes wetter and as ovulation nears you release a slippery secretion, similar to sperm.

Many people feel sexier around the time they ovulate. For many women the second week of the month is the most interesting sexually for them and produces red-hot orgasms. After ovulation, next comes the influence of progesterone which turns your mucus sticky and creamy, literally plugging

the cervix so any
implantation can
happen in peace.
As you approach
your period, the
vagina becomes more
acidic and itchy and
more prone to infections
(especially yeast), so this is
the time where you might enjoy
sex the least.

Keep an 'arousal' diary. Once a day, insert a finger into your
vagina and check the moisture levels. Are you dry, wet,
creamy or slippery? Now compare your sexual activities. Did
the changes in your vaginal environment affect your sexual
enjoyment? If you can find a link, you'll be jumping over
yourself to schedule sex activity when you are most
receptive.

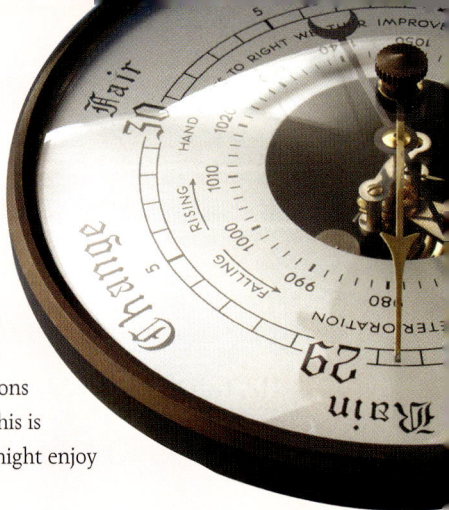

4

Myth world

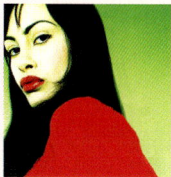

Don't let pictures of the beautiful and famous make you feel inadequate.

Even the most beautiful women can have problems feeling confident. Halle Berry is a former Miss Teen All America, was the runner-up to Miss USA and has been voted into *People* magazine's Most Beautiful People list nine times: oh, and she's also an Oscar winner. Despite all this, she recently announced that she is very insecure about both her physical appearance and her acting. Beauty is skin deep. There's no point in thinking that you would feel/be sexier if you looked different; confidence comes from within.

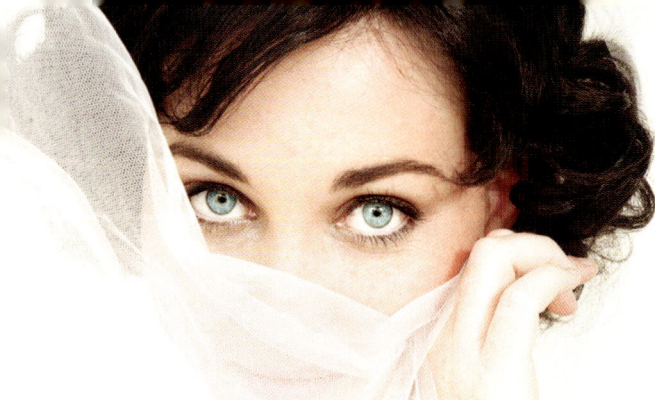

In *Hot Monogamy* Dr Patricia Love uses research that shows women who have a negative body image are 'less interested in making love ... more restricted in their range of sexual activities, and have more difficulty becoming aroused and reaching orgasm.' You have to feel sexy to have a better love life, rather than focusing on how you look. If you like, you can continue to feel down on yourself but it's better not to waste all that energy: concentrate instead on getting that orgasm high.

Get some glamorous photographs taken of you (if necessary by a professional) and keep a few of them, framed, in your bedroom. This is to remind you that you are sexy, and the better the photo the more confidence you'll feel. After all, glam shots in magazines are hardly simple snapshots!

5

Slippery when wet

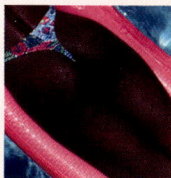

Don't think of foreplay as prelude to penetration, savour it as the main event. Go on, push the boat out!

Play around a little and find out what gets your partner off. Get your partner to talk dirty to you, moan more or indicate with their hands which spots feel good and, likewise, point him in the right direction. Don't be afraid to lend a hand and play with yourself in front of him, too.

Rubbing yourself against his hard crotch through your jeans can feel magnificent, and when he touches your naked pussy it'll feel better if you're already hot. Before you get to naked

genital contact, try kissing,
light touches (with fingertips
or feathers) and breast and
neck play. He could try cupping
your genitals with one hand
whilst the other presses on your
pubic bone. If you like oral sex, try
it in different positions; for instance,
receiving it whilst in the doggy
position feels completely different to
lying on your back. If your partner is
licking/kissing you, he can also try varying
from hot/cold temperatures or sucking a
mint or cough lozenge, all of which will
change how his tongue feels.

Hang a sheet up in the middle of a room (or
from a coat hanger on your wardrobe door)
and stand either side of it so that you can't see
each other. Naked, feel for each other through
the sheet and rub lightly up against each
other. What you think about during this, I'll
leave to you. The novelty of the experience
should make you feel aroused more quickly.

6

Shivering with anticipation

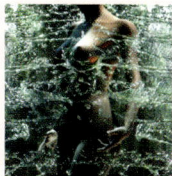

Learn how to think 'dirty'

If you're having problems getting going, think back and remember a time when you had great sex and try to get into that mindset. Try to put yourself on the couch and think about what situations are erotic for you.

Another trick is to devote a little time to just thinking about sexy thoughts: for instance, giving yourself a chance to daydream, browse erotica and the freedom to respond to sexual imagery. In a Xandria.com article, Betty Dodson suggests we tap into aural pleasure because we've been conditioned to climax and have sex silently. She recommends recording an orgasm with a tape recorder/dictaphone and playing it back; you'll probably find it's more subdued than you realise. Just practising coming in a louder, sexier way can help to free your inhibitions.

Lovers should spend time talking, thinking, imagining and revelling in each other's possibilities before moving on to manual techniques. It really is a question of mind over matter!

Get into the habit of writing down your dreams. When you go to sleep, think erotic thoughts and hopefully you'll have raunchy dreams all night – which will mean you'll wake up feeling wet and ready for a bit of love. The more you can train yourself to think sexy at odd times, like when you're waiting in a supermarket queue, the faster you'll be able to perform when it really counts.

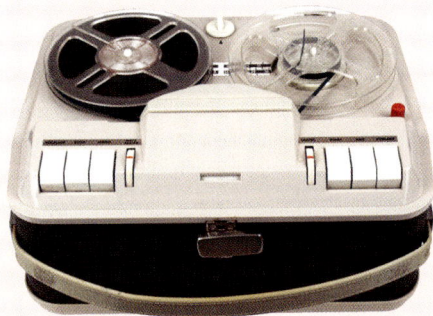

7

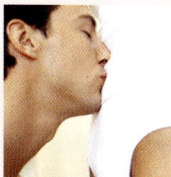

Get him to use his mouth

Being able to enjoy oral sex, as a starter or an act in itself, is a good way to ensure you have satisfying orgasms.

Many women find it easier to come this way than during penetrative sex. If you already know what tongue techniques you like best, indicate this to your partner by licking his hand in the same motion. Lie down on your back, preferably at the end of a sofa or on a bed with a pillow under your bum. Use your hands to guide your partner's head.

When you are fully stimulated, you may be ready for direct action on the clitoris. It has an astonishing 8000 nerve endings despite having no real job or function, so it can be a bit intense. Nifty tongue circles around it work well, so get your partner to try figures of eight, and playful flicks in an up and down or left to right movement. Some women like the tongue to dart in and out of the vagina, others like a finger in the vagina or anus while the clitoris is being attended to. This heightens the sexual feeling because the pleasure areas overlap. Some clitorises are more sensitive on one side; use your other mouth to scream where. It should feel amazing by now!

Treat yourself to a pair of real silk undies and get your partner to spend as long as possible licking you through the material before he gets to your clit. When you've been teased and tingled for a while you'll be screaming for more.

8

Starter's orders

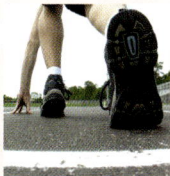

Ways to slow down the pace and get your partner to be more touchy-feely...

Men often dive right in to genital play because that's what they prefer, but if you're into some romantic kissing first, followed by breast fondling, then simply keep kissing him until he gets the message and slow foreplay down to a tempo that you're comfortable with. If you're already naked and he's too eager, try one of the tips from the *Kama Sutra* – the Biting of a Boar. He sits on his haunches and you sit between his knees with your back to him. He can kiss or lightly bite (or breathe on) your back, shoulders and neck.

If he's prone to premature ejaculation or just too impatient, another approach is to get him to have a quick climax first so that he'll be able to focus on pleasing you. I once heard of a fetish club where each man received a blow job when he got through the door so he could properly enjoy the night's proceedings. If you don't feel like doing this, you can encourage him to masturbate, or do it for him using lots of lube. This will mechanically slow him down for his next orgasm because his seminal vesicle and prostate need time to create more seminal fluid.

Ask your partner to give you some time alone to get in the mood, anything from ten to thirty minutes, but don't agree on what time he should come in and disturb you. Start to masturbate; the fact that you don't know when to expect him will add to your tension. Let him catch you playing with yourself, and when he sees what you're up to you should be already nicely aroused.

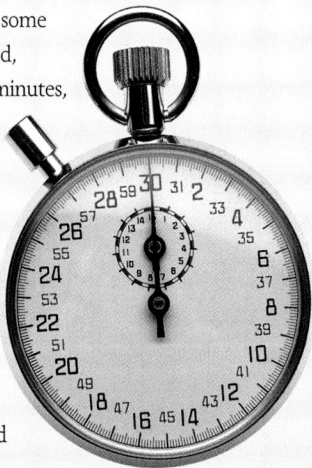

9

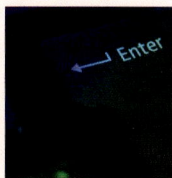

Point of entry

Daring ways to take the lead in seduction and try a bit of role bending!

Try focusing on his bits for a change and ask him to guide your hand in the right direction. Getting him to open up to what feels good is an excellent way to learn how to read each other's needs. See if he likes having his nipples played with and put an exploratory finger in his mouth to get him used to the feeling of being penetrated. This is all gentle stuff to get him used to the idea.

An ingenious device to assist with positioning is getting a 'love swing' fixed to the ceiling. This allows you to try a greater range of positions at angles that are just not possible lying on a bed. You can both sit on it, or one of you can lie spread-eagled, or hang tantalisingly over the edge. It also swings and bounces when you have sex and the movement intensifies the rhythm of your strokes. If you position your man on a love swing, you will increase his sense of helplessness.

Take it in turns to take command of who does what in your lovemaking. When it's your turn, try something different and see if you can roll around from one position to the next. You can also choose a new position from fun websites like www.sexualpositionsfree.com – it uses only dolls in various poses, so you won't find it shocking.

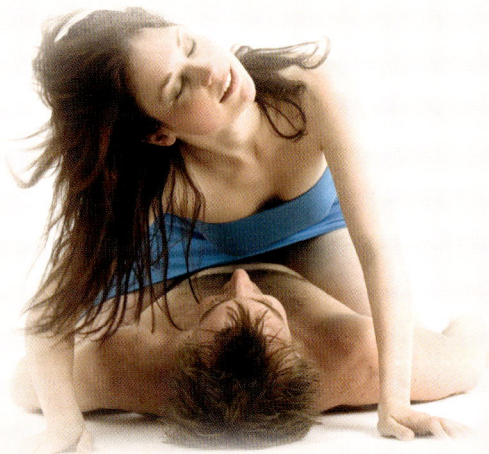

10

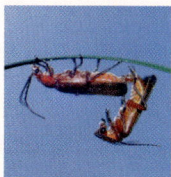

Classic positions

These classic sexual moves
are here to stay, so make
the most of them and modify
them slightly for a little
diversity...

Couples who experiment generally have a sexual repertoire that
includes a couple of basic positions, and these are likely to be the
missionary and woman on top. It's often easier to begin sex play
with missionary because with the woman prone on her back and
the man's weight supported on his knees, it's an easier vantage
point to actually insert the penis.

Both men and women generally find it easier to come when they're on top, and if you're pregnant or nervous about the depth of the penetration, being in control means that you take charge of the strokes. You can lie down over your partner, balancing your weight forward onto your clitoris and you're in an ideal position to use your knees to rock, thrust or push your way to orgasm. You can also sit up (note that you get better penetration if you do this sitting on a chair with no arms so your legs can use the floor for leverage) and just choose to rock back and forth. A variation is to lean back more, still straddling his penis so your clitoris is exposed, making it dead easy for you to play with it and giving him a ringside seat. Another trick is for you to sit the other way facing his feet reverse 'cowgirl' style, which gives you a different feeling again and is ideal for men who worship an exposed *derriere* in action.

11

The long and short of it

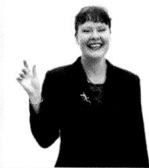

It's not just about how long, how hard and how thick

We're an average lot. The Lifestyles Condom Penis Size survey measured 300 stiff penises and concluded (amazingly) that 82% of women were content with an average-sized penis of about 6 inches. Conveniently, it just so happens the average erect love stick is 5.9 inches and its girth 5 inches. Only 2% of women wanted an extra-large penis (over 10 inches, like you see in porn films) and only 9% a bigger-than-average penis (7–8 inches).

If you want more sensation, some positions are better suited for a smaller to average willy. The missionary position is improved with a pillow under the woman's bottom. Even

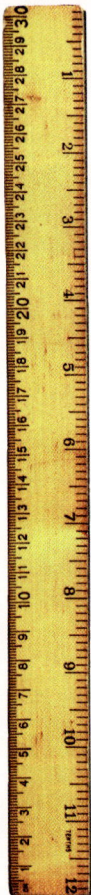

better, if you can, bend your legs back and hook them around his neck. Crossing your ankles in this position helps to tighten the vaginal canal. You'll also find that woman on top positions work well, especially if you sit on a chair so you have more leverage. Other favourites are doggy style (although some men report falling out); here the best thing is for the man to use his hands to hold the woman's bum and control both thrusts. Others swear by the scissor position, lying with your heads in opposite directions, 'scissoring' your legs with each other's (one of you has a leg underneath the other) and with you facing him in a sideways twist, holding hands.

For a fuller feeling, try using an anal plug whilst having sex. This will help to shorten the vaginal opening because your perineum (the bit in the middle between your vagina and anus) is being pulled in two different directions. Kind of naughty but nice, it will also feel like you're having two men at once!

12

Larging it

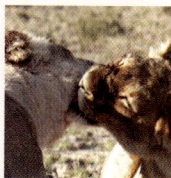

There's nothing acrobatic or difficult about the CAT and you could improve your chances of having an orgasm with it by up to 50%!

The CAT (Coitally Adjusted Technique) was 'invented' in the 1990s in America and it's specifically designed for extra clitoral stimulation. You start off in the basic missionary position, but your partner should rest his full weight on your chest and you should manoeuvre until you're lying with both pelvic bones touching. This way he's riding higher than normal (his head will be around 15 cm further up the bed), most of his penis is out of your vagina, but the head of it is pressing alluringly against your *cli-cli*. You should wrap your legs around him as this allows him to penetrate you more deeply and you're going to need to hold on tightly to each other. Now you both rock together, keeping your pelvises tight against each other, avoiding thrusting movements: there's no in and out action with this one. The idea is to rock gently to a climax. Women have 50% more chance of climaxing in this position, and the non-thrusting aspect of it makes him less likely to come. It's also a good position for coming at the same time.

Try creating your own new sex position. Experiment with postures and try moving your legs, and pelvis differently for a better fit. The dominant person should try different ways of supporting their hands – higher, lower and prone on the body. Both of you have a go at being on top and see whether you prefer to lean forwards (for clitoral stimulation) or backwards to nudge your G-spot.

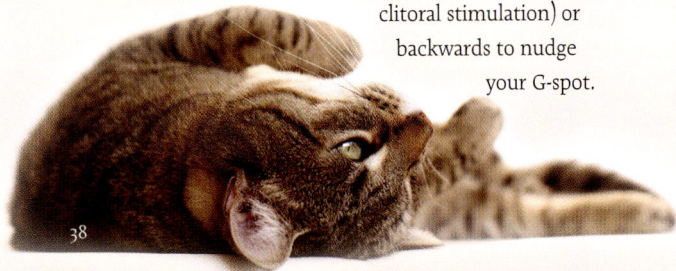

13

Toys R no fuss

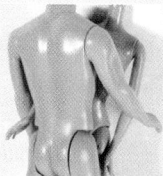

You can use vibrators all over your body or dive in and cut to the chase.

More than half of couples use some form of sex aid to spice up their sex life and manufacturers are now producing insertable vibrators and dildos that are curved to match the natural shape of the vagina and rectum. You do need to experiment to find out what materials and shapes appeal to you. If you don't feel comfortable about self-insertion, try a clitoral massager like the Fun Factory Layaspot which simply sits over your pubic bone and hums away; it has different speeds and programmes to vary the tempo. You can also keep it in place whilst have sex with your partner (he'll share a bit of the thrill too).

The first time you insert a sex toy, don't feel a pressure to put it all in. You're more sensitive on the outer third of your vagina, so some women like to just nudge and stimulate this area. If your partner is using a toy on you, he can start by performing cunnilingus and then inserting a finger or two until you're ready, but always go slow and insert just a little. The time for shoving it in is when you're screaming with pleasure!

Try masturbating with more than one sex toy. You can use a dildo/vibrator in your vagina and combine this with a vibrator tickling your clitoris (or Vielle's finger gloves). If you really want to push the boat out, you can use an anal plug as well. You stand more chance of having better orgasms if you have more than one area being stimulated.

14

Alternative erogenous zones

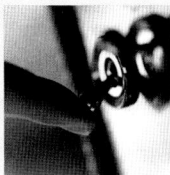

In a long-term relationship it's useful to continue finding new areas to make meaningful to your lover, and anal play is something you could both potentially enjoy.

If you'd like to try anal play, get your partner to give you really good foreplay first and get you warmed up. It's best to test the perineum first; if this feels nice being massaged, then you'll probably want some anal touch too. Get your partner to use lots of lubricant and to just use a finger to gently probe the area. You can also lick it too (known as rimming).

Start with a finger or small butt plug first. Use lots of lube and take it slow. At first it may feel strange, but after the initial opening, it quickly becomes accommodating and pleasurable.

For full anal penetrative sex, forget what you see on porn videos. Use lots of lube (the anus has no natural lubrication). The most difficult part is initially getting the penis in there. It's best if you find a position where you can control entry with your hands (get him to push gently) so that he enters you at the right angle in some kind of comfort zone. When it's comfortable, he can increase the pace. Don't forget to top up on lube as you go along and stop if it starts to hurt. In the throes of passion, you might not notice any discomfort so remember it's how you feel *afterwards* that's the real indicator of any soreness factor. Many women find it easier to come through anal penetration when they are on top because it stimulates the clitoris. It's also a different type of orgasm, so play around a little, and find your next big thing.

15

Hot spots

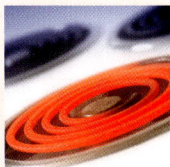

If the clitoris doesn't do it for you, simply experiment and find out what tickles your fancy.

The next time you take a shower do an internal examination. About three inches inside the vagina you're likely to find a spongy spot about the shape of an almond. If you can't locate it try taking a pee, and you should be able to feel the urine moving through the vaginal wall. Remember, it's not *on* the wall, probe and feel for it *through* the wall.

You can add another dimension to your love life by opting to stimulate it more. When you masturbate, go for both clitoral and vaginal stimulation, using a finger or special curved dildo to touch the spot. If someone is going down on you, get them to insert a finger/s and touch you inside as well. Hitting both spots should produce deeper, more intense contractions. For penetration, you might want to experiment with positions that work the G-spot more, such as woman on top and rear entry.

Other hot spots include the U-spot (the sensitive opening to the urethra), the X-spot on the cervix and what the sex therapist Barbara Keesling calls 'tenting' – the area behind the cervix which lifts up during sex to allow penetration of the space behind. Finally, find out if your G spot is sensitive before having a hysterectomy – if it is, you can have a supra-cervical operation where they leave the cervix in. You don't want to find out too late!

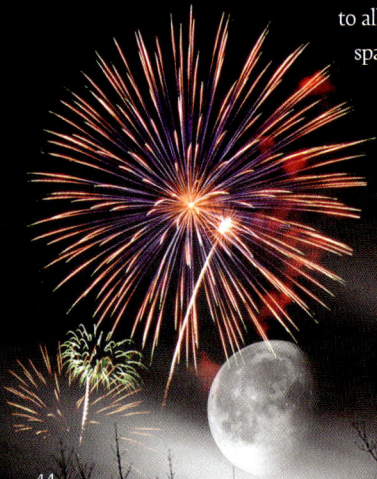

16

Ride the wave

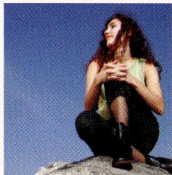

Here are some simple techniques to make you insatiable

There are two types of multiple orgasms. Sequential multiples come close together (two to ten minutes apart); the classic way is for a woman to come through oral sex and then to follow this with another during penetrative sex. A wilder ride is serial multiple orgasms which come right after each other like a roller-coaster ride. This occurs when all the hot spots are being stimulated (preferably more than two at once) and the best position is woman on top because you have more control. Of course, you should also be prepared to lend yourself a hand and to stimulate your clitoris/anus or alternative erogenous zone with your hand or vibrator.

Another technique, 'peaking', plays with your arousal level. Barbara Keesling says 'As you make love, note your arousal levels on a scale from 1 to 10, with 10 being orgasm. As you reach each level, briefly stop and allow your arousal to subside so that, rather than shooting for the moon, your arousal rides in a wave-like pattern.' You can also fool your body into coming with another technique – 'plateauing' – where you mimic some of the physical aspects of orgasm by squeezing your PC muscles, speeding up your breathing and tensing your arm or leg muscles. Keesling claims you can train your body into responding to climax effortlessly at will. It's really a question of keeping going, experimenting and devoting far more time to enjoying all of your pleasure zones!

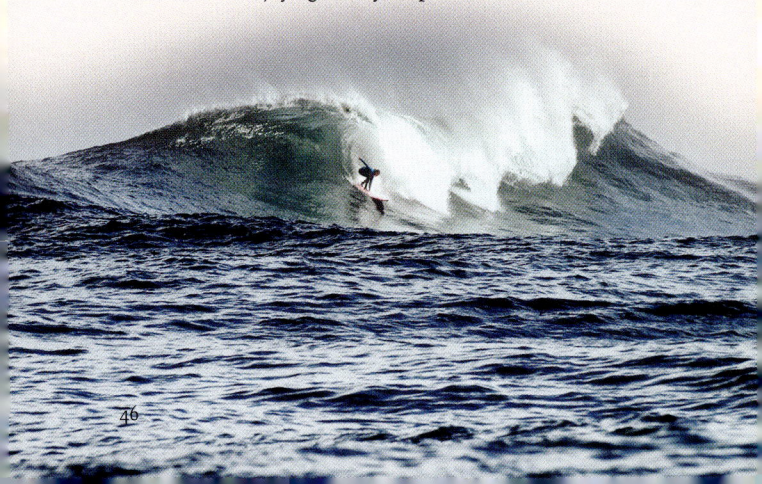

17

Giving it some

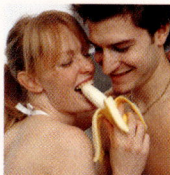

Here's how to drive your man
wild — put a few tricks up
your sleeve

Talk dirty to him, and let him see as much of your body as
possible. Men are much more receptive to sight and smell, so
if you want to give him a handjob, do it so he can see your
excited vagina. It's less work if you use lubricant on your
hands – his penis will automatically bump up and down, so
use pressure that feels good for him. The most sensitive part
of the penis is the frenulum (where the head meets the
shaft) so stimulate this especially well. One technique is to
keep one hand on the penis at all times stroking its head
(preferably slick with lube) while your other hand gives long
strokes to the rest of his penis.

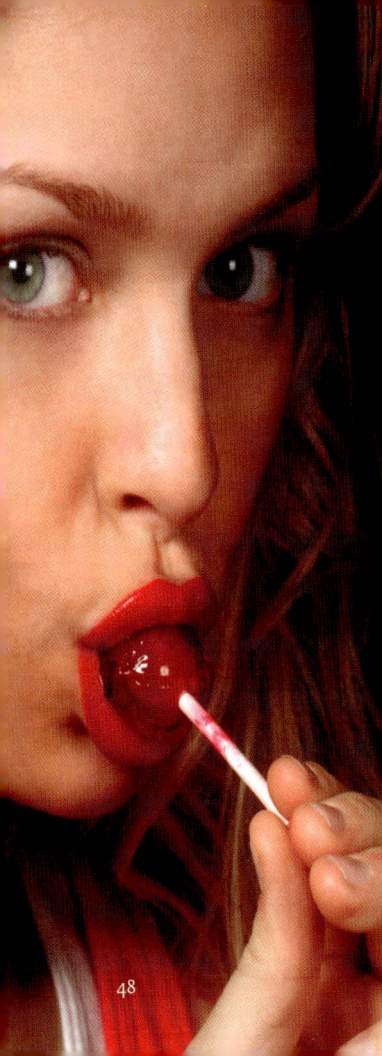

Men love oral sex. To increase his pleasure tie your hair back so he can see you doing it; even better, do it on your knees so that he can cop an eyeful of your breasts and extended neck. Brush your lips against his head, tickle him with your tongue and vary the sucking strokes.

Kneading the testicles works well, particularly the seam of it which contains lots of nerve endings. Some men can orgasm just from prostate stimulation, the male G-spot, which is just inside the anus. You could probe this with a finger or insert a well-greased butt-plug, but check first if he's game.

"Sex is like money;
only too much
is enough"

JOHN UPDIKE

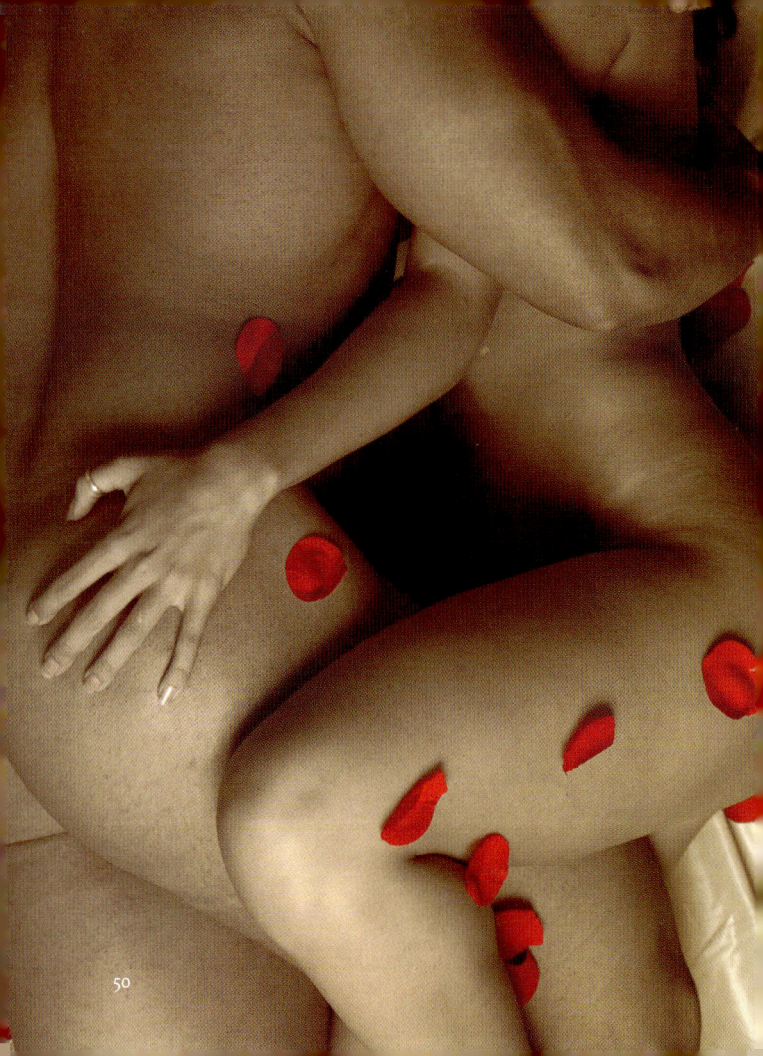

18

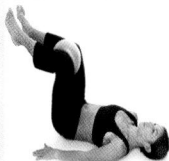

Sexercise

It's not just your bum that you need to tone up... Simple fitness tips to pep up your stamina and sort you out for the long haul

Any exercise is good for you, but the optimum way to achieve better orgasms is to strengthen and tighten your pelvic floor – the actual muscles that do the most work during sex. This is the group of six muscles that control and hold in place all of the holes in that area: the urethra, vagina and anus. In modern life we sit rather than squat, so often these muscles are weakened. Regular 'love squeezes' tighten and tone the muscles, a sure-fire way to put the zip back into your love life!

You've probably heard of Kegel exercises. They were designed to offset the problems of urinary incontinence, especially in pregnant women, but the bonus side effect is a tightened, toned vagina. The best way to find your PC muscles is to put a finger in your vagina and clench your muscles. You should be able to feel pressure on your finger. Very often, people use the wrong muscles, so have a few goes until you feel something. Try more fingers or a dildo if you're having difficulty. Once you've found your muscles, clench them, and try to clench your anus, vagina and urethra muscles separately. Clench and release. Try to do ten contractions, have a rest and go for ten more. Breathe evenly throughout. When you've got the hang of it, try to do them every day or as often as you can manage.

19

Tell it like it is

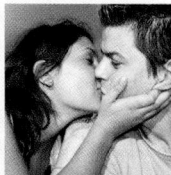

Let the cat out of the bag
and express yourself to lovers,
in your diary or under a nom
de plume on the net.

Talking is easy when things are going right. The problems
start when things get jaded, or go downhill. To get you in the
mood for talking frankly, you could watch a film about sex
(erotic or otherwise) to make the subject easier to discuss. If
you can't bring yourself to watch anything erotic yet, talk
about a couple in any film that features modern
relationships.

There are also emails, texting, phone calls and journals. Some people find it easier to talk dirty over a phone because they can let their guard down without having to reveal their body language. Another tip is to write down your ideal fantasy and leave it somewhere your lover can read it. Make it sizzling hot, just how you'd like it to happen.

Ask your lover to tell you a story; it can be anything. But once you've established this, ask him to tell you about his first sexual experience, or the first time he had sex with you. Work up to him confessing his 'fantasy' story with all the bits and bobs he never normally reveals.

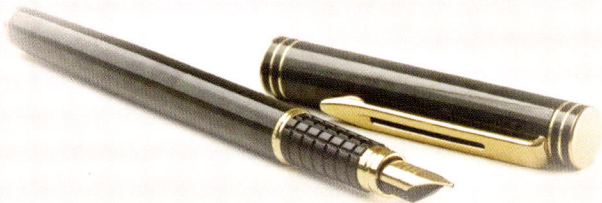

20

Mind games

Not enough hours in the day? Too tired? The most erotic place is the mind, so role play and snatch back time to salvage those precious moments...

One of the advantages of being in a long-term relationship is that you get to know how the other person ticks. Even if you're not conscious of it, you've built up a system of codes, rituals and associations that instantly signals your mood. For instance, if you're into playing with ice cubes during foreplay, a seemingly innocuous glass filled with ice takes on a whole different meaning. There's a lot of mileage to be gained from playing out your fantasies.

Common sexual fantasies that couples role play involve power dynamics such as master and pupil, nurse and patient, and being taken against your will. Other scenarios might be that you're a virgin or meeting for the first time: it's really your call.

To act out a fantasy, first of all you have to find out what turns you on and work out your boundaries. (If you want to walk all over him with high-heeled shoes, it could be he insists you throw a rug over him first.) Perhaps you want to eroticise things you find not so good, like a Caesarean scar or needing to have safe sex. The delicious thing about head play is that you can talk over the details first at length and use this to get each other off. You might want to invest in some props to make it more authentic. For women, a wig and certain types of shoes and/or underwear are very effective, and it's a great excuse to play around with make-up, temporary tattoos and accessories. Just like making a film, you come up with a script, work out the characters, sets and costumes, and then set it up so it's ready to roll.

21

Compromise positions

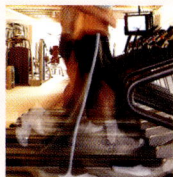

Ways to satisfy each other when you don't have time to go all the way

It's all very well waxing lyrical about leisurely techniques, but sometimes we just don't have time to put them into practice. A lot of us would rather catch up on shut-eye instead. However, sleepy lovers can improvise to speed things along. To get you warmed up, try starting foreplay earlier whilst you are watching TV and then you can finish off in the bedroom. If one of you showers at night join them and have sex right there in the shower – one of the best positions for couples in a hurry is to do it standing up, and this way there's no need to clean up afterwards. If he's not up to penetrating you, you can buy a dildo to stick on the shower wall for you to ride on and give him a full view.

Other tricks involve making use of new technology to get you aroused quicker. The Tantra Beam massager (tantrabeam.com) is an electric pulse device you wear on your wrist like a watch; the strap slips over your finger. You're still touching your partner with the feel of your own skin, but when you switch on the machine it literally electrifies your touch which makes for a quick thrill. (To really push the boat out, he can wear this around his waist and turn his penis into a vibrator.) It's also good as a relaxing massager if you just want a bit of touchy-feely. In your regular lovemaking sessions make a mental list of things that turn each other on and discover positions that make you come quicker for maximum effect (both men and women generally find it easier to come on top).

22

Seeing is believing

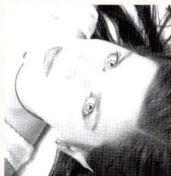

Doing something as simple as looking at each other properly during foreplay and sex can increase intimacy and give you 'full-bodied' orgasms

Literal 'love making', with lots of eye contact and tenderness, heightens the connection between you and your partner. You might want to start by looking at your partner more when he's naked. Chat to him when he's in the bath or shower. Learn the little gestures, like the small hand and facial movements he makes, so that you can read his expressions.

Once you have this intimacy, you'll know how to read him the next time you get flirty. Find out what things turn him on (does he like lacy undies, stockings, leather, a hair-free zone?) and get him to wear those things that please you.

The missionary position is the classic one for keeping lip and eye contact, but there are other face-to-face positions that feel more personal. The Fitter-In has both of you sitting facing each other with your legs over his hips. Grip each other's arms and rock in position and connect with your eyes. For even cosier variations, sit up in his lap (still facing each other) with your legs around his back. All these positions allow you to cuddle, caress, and look lovingly into each other's eyes as well as have sex.

Try making love in positions where you spend more time gazing into each other's eyes. The Inverted Embrace from the Kama Sutra is ideal. The woman is on top, and lies prone against the man's chest, pressing her breasts to his body, then she moves her hands down to grip his hips. With your upper body flat down, you can rock to orgasm and exchange loving glances all the way.

23

Sex in water

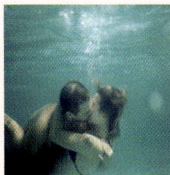

The versatility of water makes it the ideal medium for adding the X factor to your sex life.

Of course, it's not so easy to literally have sex in water. If you're lucky enough to have your own whirlpool or private swimming pool, this makes life easier, although keep a tube of silicone lube nearby as penetrative sex in water tends to wash away your natural moisture.

These days, there are loads of waterproof sex toys that help you to get off discreetly. For instance, you could insert Fun Factory pleasure balls and then go for a swim in your local pool or sit in a spa. There's also the Wireless Waterproof Vibrating Panty with a wireless waterproof micro-orb that fits into the pants. Wear a swimsuit over it and nobody will notice.

Alternatively, there are plenty of bath and shower accessories that can be put to good use. Almost every type of sex toy imaginable comes in a waterproof version and you can get dildo accessories to stick on the shower door or side of the bath. Some toys look perfectly innocuous: for instance, there's a Sponge vibrator that gets you clean as well, and a Ducky vibrator that gets going when you give the little fellow a squeeze.

If you don't like the idea of sticking something inside you, the Layaspot clitoris massager from the Fun Factory is perfect for you. It's waterproof and has a range of vibrations and fits snugly over the pubic bone. Simply lie back and relax and let the machine do the work. Mmm…

24

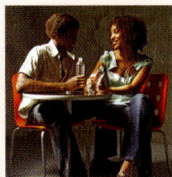

Dangerous liaisons

Flirting boosts your self-esteem and is uplifting. Even if it's just harmless fun, it's sure to put a spring in your step.

Flirting is simply about feeling upbeat, smiling and using body language that conveys positive emotions. The crucial way to flirt is to use your eyes more. If you're in a social situation, glance around the room and let your eyes linger on the people you find interesting. Be careful, though, as eye contact is such a powerful way to communicate.

Pay careful attention to your posture. Don't cross your arms or use body parts to block off your partner; adopting an open, confident smiling posture makes you seem easier to talk to. Keep your back straight and avoid hunching your shoulders; it makes you seem more outgoing – and makes you look slimmer too!

Do flirt with people who you stand a chance of getting somewhere with. Striving to get someone's sexual interest and exploring the possibilities of 'will we, won't we' is what it's all about. You never know where that spark of passion will lead…

The next time you're at a social gathering with your partner, pick out the most attractive man in the room and make a point of talking to him animatedly. It's harmless fun, you're aiming to boost your self-confidence, and if you have a lover in tow it'll show him there could be a little competition….

25

Sexpert advice

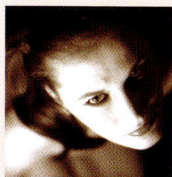

Porn star Stormy Daniels gives us the low-down on her job, her love life and her top sex tips

Stormy has been working in feature porn films since 2004. She doesn't work in front of the cameras every day; she also dances, writes and directs porn films.

A porn shoot is two to four days of filming and the actors have less sex than you might think. Stormy may actually only have forty minutes of penetrative sex. The sex scenes aren't scripted and if you're wondering how the actresses seem to be instantly horny, this is because they get about an hour and a half of foreplay during the lead-in: tell your partner you want to be treated like a porn star and demand the same!

She doesn't pre-lubricate herself beforehand and says to get herself psyched up she'll go and watch scenes being filmed. The hair and make-up preparation also helps too. You might not really feel like having sex that much but if you pamper yourself a bit you'll be more open to the idea. Stormy suggests that if you feel beautiful before you have sex, you're more likely to enjoy yourself.

Her advice to women looking to be a bit more orgasmic is 'Have sex with yourselves to find out what you like. Speak up and say what you want and experiment in bed. If women stop having sex, they stop craving it. But once you get started, the more sex you have, the more you want it.'

26

Be contrary

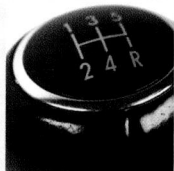

Being intimate is a double-edged sword. Sometimes it brings you too close and you need to be a bit more sexually ruthless to enjoy getting off.

If your sex life is nothing to write home about, try deliberately avoiding it for a while. If something's on tap you take it for granted. See how long you can go without having sex together. It's a good idea not to stop all physical activity: you could try masturbating separately and telling each other all about it when you do get together. You could also try playing around with sexual fantasy. Get him to dress up a little differently or speak to you in bed in a different voice.

Now's the time to inject some throbbing desire into the proceedings. It could be that he's treating you gently when you really want to be ravaged, so try talking dirty and see if this makes it easier for you to get excited. Force yourself to expose your throbbing desires. That's it – get low and dirty and sex up your relationship.

Ask your partner to describe your contribution to your lovemaking; make a careful note of what he says, then for a limited time reverse this behaviour. If he normally initiates sex, you do it for a change. You'll have sex sessions using completely different methods and techniques to the ones you're used to, and perhaps you'll be pleasantly surprised!

27

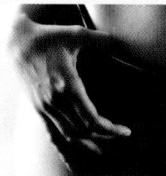

Indecent proposal

Fantasising is normal human behaviour. Once you've worked out what makes you tick, you've got a fast-track route to orgasms

Women think about sex at least four and a half times a day. The trick is to hold on to some of these fleeting images so you can make use of them. Keep a dream/mood diary, and note down things and people that arouse a flicker of sexual interest. The trick is to find out what turns you on. Try browsing websites like www.cliterati.co.uk or www.literotic.com. Some women find their wildest thoughts are actually quite mundane. Don't worry if your fantasy isn't exotic, as the most common one is sex with a current or past lover.

Try to spend some time in the week on your own, safe behind a locked door. Some find sanctuary in the bathroom, where they can sip a glass of wine as they soak in the bath and let their mind wander. Let your thoughts take you wherever they want to go, and resist the urge to self-censor. The next step is masturbation. Ideally you've titillated yourself with erotic thoughts first, as once your body has responded and you are moist it's easier to play with yourself. The joint action of fantasising and masturbation is a double turn-on.

To delve deeper into his sexual psyche, get your partner to write his secret fantasies on your back with a lip liner pencil. You won't be able to see them unless you look in a mirror (and then you have to be able to read backwards) so his secret is safe unless he can trust you enough to reveal all. If you only get part of the way in one session, have a bath and get him to wash it all off.

28

Fancy a Brazilian?

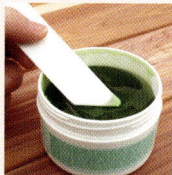

The jury's out on whether it's better for your bush to be au naturel or not.

Whatever you do, do it to increase your sexual confidence and to boost your body image. Ring the changes and you'll feel more sexually confident. If you want to depilate for a V shape, you could consider the common methods: a bikini line wax, shaving or a depilation cream. It's best to have waxing done at a salon but you will need at least six weeks' growth. It is painful (avoid doing it when you are premenstrual and feel pain more intensely) but it will be smooth for around four weeks. Avoid having a bath or shower after waxing, and exfoliate with a loofah or body scrub every few days to prevent a rash as the hairs start to come back.

To remove more of the hair, or the whole lot, you could try a Brazilian wax or shaving. It's best to have a Brazilian done at a speciality salon; it will take around half an hour and all the parts of your vulva, including your anus, will be waxed.

You can also shave yourself at home. It's best to soften the hair first by having a bath, or lying a wet cloth over it. Use conditioner on your pubic hair to pre-soften. Cut the hair short with scissors or with an electric beard trimmer. (First timers might want to try an overall trim first to see how it feels – I promise this will not prickle the skin.) Other methods include laser surgery, which needs repeated sessions, sugaring and threading. Ask your beautician about these.

29

Dosing up

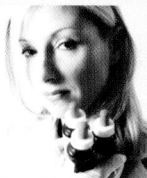

What can you do to pep up a flagging libido?

Since 1998 we've had Viagra. It can work wonders for men, but it doesn't do so much for women. Viagra is not a sexual stimulant; it works by helping to increase the blood flow – a godsend in certain sensitive areas, but it's probably effective for only one in ten women.

For the more practical, there are also rubbing lotions like L-arginine amino-acid cream which is reputed to give better arousal and orgasm. Some women swear by testosterone therapy. A new trend in cosmetic surgery is plumping up the G-spot with injections. Devotees say it increases sensations, but it has to be done every few months, so I hope it's worth the effort!

An American surgeon has developed an electronic spinal implant which makes use of neurally augmented surgery to implant an electrode into the spinal area that attaches to a device, the orgasmatron, which stimulates orgasm. In tests, women who had never had an orgasm were able to experience one. The treatment costs $17,000 and only one person in the world is currently offering this service. A temporary one-week implant costs $3,800 and makes for a romantic vacation; for more details see www.aipmnc.com.

Try Femi-X, the new exciting product from Medic House. The multi-pack contains herbal tablets designed to naturally increase female libido, and it comes complete with an educational CD and a cool DVD featuring clitoris-friendly positions. It's available at pharmacies or from www.femi-x.com.

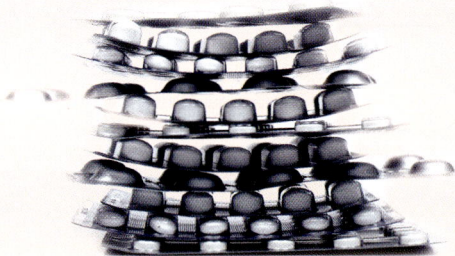

30

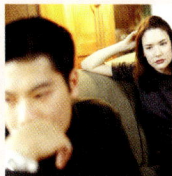

Coming back after turning off

If you just never feel in the mood any more, reconnecting with your sexual self is the first stage.

In certain situations it's normal to 'go off' sex. If you've not been enjoying the sex you've been having, or if it's become painful or emotionally strained, it's only natural that you're not going to be queuing up to repeat the experience. The good news is that it's exactly when you're in this take it or leave it cul-de-sac that you have the restraint necessary to pick up some new moves and techniques.

Go back to basics and initiate sessions devoted exclusively to foreplay. Leave your clothes on and fool around. Talk and snuggle up with your partner whenever you can. Grab the opportunity to find out if something about your sexual tastes has changed. If the vaginal area is sore or out of bounds, try responding to breast, anal or foot fondling instead. Touching, kissing, hugging and stroking are all just as good as sex (ask a foot fetishist!).

Trust yourself and give yourself time to enjoy anything that comes your way. Take a warm bath, pop in a bath bomb, lie back and put on a face pack and drink lots of fresh juices as you chill out in scented water. You'll be less stressed (a libido buster) and the warm water improves blood circulation and gets things moving more quickly. Try masturbating with your shower spray or a waterproof dildo on your clit; a very clean way to get horny.

31

Your sexual profile

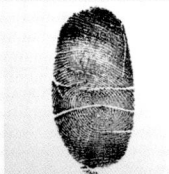

Do you have a 'template' that traces your sexual predilections?

Given that first-time sex can be a bit hit and miss, it's a little scary to think that this can affect our whole perception of sex for years to come. What we think of as our personal sexual predilections are probably inherited from a formative sexual blueprint. This makes a good argument for choosing a good man for the job, but for many of us it's too late; we have to live with our blueprints. If you look hard at what was imprinted into you that first couple of times, you'll find you've been unconsciously replicating this. Did he turn you on to rough sex? What's your preferred way to kiss? This is especially important because if you've had a bad experience you may have been avoiding things that could give you pleasure with the right partner.

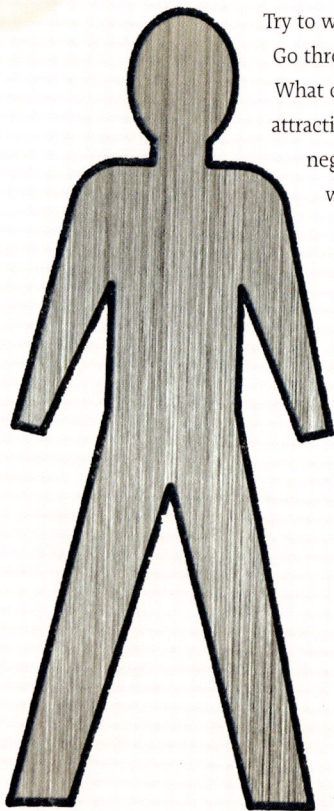

Try to work out your sexual template. Go through old photos of your lovers. What characteristics do you find attractive? Now think about what negative traits these lovers brought with them. If you could go back in time, what things would you change? Mentally revise your checklist. It could be that over time you go for the security of someone in gainful employment rather than a wannabe rock star.

32

Let yourself go

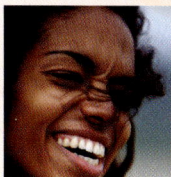

Challenge yourself to lose one of your inhibitions.

People who are shy are not necessarily suffering from low self-esteem. They behave that way because they're overly concerned with their self-image. If you're feeling nervous about not being able to come you can counter this by focusing on your partner's pleasure, the music that's playing, the beautiful sunset, whatever. Stop thinking of yourself as a spectator and just go with the flow; at a nightclub if you thought consciously of all the moves you were making whilst dancing, you'd stop yourself from moving. Let your body fall into its own rhythm or choose static positions like the doggy style where you can relax and enjoy being 'done to'.

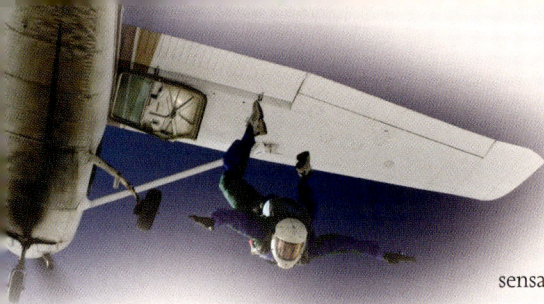

It can also help to focus on one sensation, like the feel of your hair whipping back, the movement of your skin, your partner's face. Don't be afraid to moan and do at least try to look like you're having a ball. If you think positive, you're much more likely to get the result you want. Top athletes train by visualising goals as if they were already achieved and, strangely, these mental tricks seem to work. Yep, it is possible to kid yourself into having a real orgasm.

This weekend you're going to try something daring. What about caving, riding a roller coaster, go-karting or learning to dive? Book yourself a session or a class and just go for it. If you find the experience nerve-racking at first, just imagine your sense of achievement (and relief) when you've completed it. Now think about doing the same in bed.

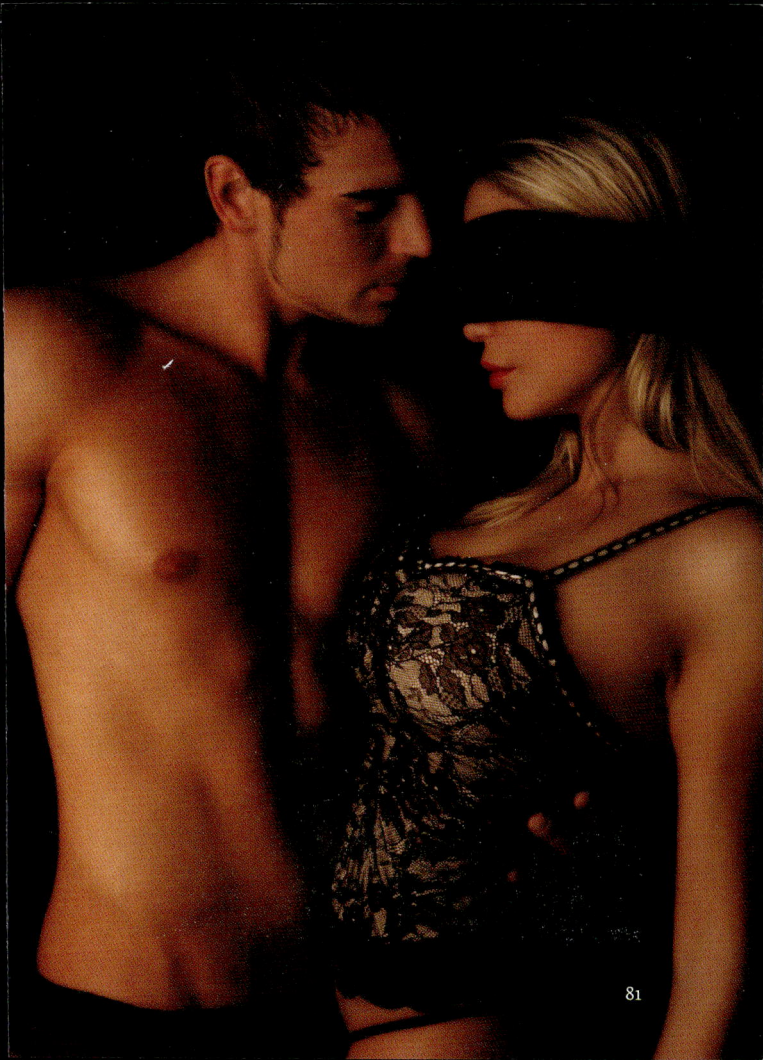

"Sex appeal is fifty per cent what you've got and fifty per cent what people think you've got"

SOPHIA LOREN

33

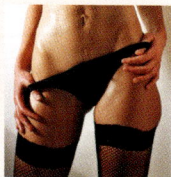

Pandora's box

A glimpse of the weird and wonderful world of pornography.

There are magazines and websites that cater for every fantasy and predilection; some get off on fetishising part of the body such as *Legs* or prefer to see women partially clad, as in *Panty Play*. It might surprise you to know that some men seek hairy, large or 'mature' women as a sexual preference and there are numerous magazines to cater for this.

Of course, there are adult magazines aimed at women too, *Scarlet, For Women* and *Playgirl* cover all aspects of erotica and feature male pin-ups; www.forthegirls.com is an erotica site with photos specially chosen for women. Lesbian magazines like *Diva* and *Curve* present female sexuality in an alternative way and often have more interesting articles. If you prefer a good read, try the *Erotic Review, Forum*, www.erotica-readers.com or my favourite, www.nerve.com, which was set up because 'sex is beautiful and absurd, remarkably fun and reliably trauma-inducing.'

Fetish magazines tend to be high quality and glossy, and less overtly in-your-face sexual. The most glamorous is *Marquis*, which features beautiful fetish fashion; *Skin Two* contains more articles around the scene and *Secret* is focused on bondage. We're still just scratching the surface but this should give you an idea of the competing ideals for what constitutes 'sexy' and what makes you hot.

Try arranging a party with your girlfriends. Along with the bottles of wine, ask everyone to bring some porn they find stimulating. By the end of the night you should have had a laugh and discovered some tantalising stuff.

34

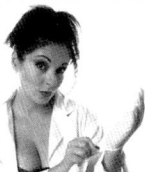

Beyond the beyond

The road to excess leads to the palace of wisdom. Tips for the sexually adventurous (not for the faint-hearted).

You might be surprised to know that what you do in the bedroom is influenced by what professional performers get up to in porn. So if you want to have wild sex like Jenna Jameson, here are some tips to help you along.

For advanced play you need new techniques. For example, instead of just penetration, you might want to experiment with fisting which is popular in the lesbian community. If you're new to it, get your partner to do it for you. He must be patient (fisting can take up to an hour) and slow, and learn to work with how much your vagina muscles can take.

Start by lubricating with a water-based lube and playing around with one finger, adding others one at a time. You have to be incredibly horny to be able to enjoy this. Using lots of stimulation and lube, get him to play with you and slowly add more fingers. See how far you can go. If he can insert four fingers, you're nearly there and it's just a question of him squashing his fingers together and twisting his hand to go further in. If it becomes uncomfortable, take some of the fingers out or stop altogether. A diagonal route is the best way to get the whole hand in.

Some women describe being fisted as the ultimate orgasm and when this happens, your muscles might clench so much they push his hand out. He has to go with the flow, but must never take his hand out quickly – it can take as long to get out as it took to get in, so this is not an activity to do in the five minutes before bedtime. If the vaginal opening forms a 'vacuum seal' around his wrist, get him to insert a finger to break 'the seal'.

35

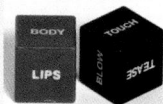

Ringing the changes

Even if it works for you, doing the same thing every time gets old

Rather than concentrating on hot new techniques, being more playful in the bedroom works wonders. For instance, you could play Twister naked, or stage a food fight: anything to get you having fun together. You can try strip poker or spin the bottle. Sites like www.mypleasure.com are teeming with erotic games to play on a rainy day. For a gentle introduction to playing at S and M, the Sensual Sweet Surrender game gives you rules and props such as a blindfold, feather, rubber tickler and flavoured massage oil. Although it's a bonus if you get turned on by these activities, don't be afraid just to mess about.

Alternatively, you can get professional and play with the Body Talk Tattoo Set which contains stencils, brushes and chocolate frosting with commands that you can temporarily paint onto the body. And then there's lick-off body gel and body finger paints for you to have fun with. And you need this sense of fun if you want to try out specifically sexual things like new positions, erogenous zones or sex toys.

If you're not that fussed about new underwear or sex toys, why not try some liquid latex? You can buy it and simply paint it on your body. It's best to shave before applying it (then it's easier to remove), and you can use it to create temporary underwear. Three coats are recommended and each takes around ten minutes to dry. After use, simply peel it off. Imagine the fun you could have decorating each other's bodies!

36

Eyes wide shut

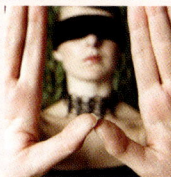

A simple blindfold can give you hours of fun, heighten your erotic potential and even doubles as a party game.

If you blindfold someone it has more of an effect than, say, changing their sense of taste. It's also one of the easiest senses to block and you can use things like a pair of tights, a scarf or even plasters under sunglasses to achieve it. You can experiment with different coloured cloth, wet blindfolds or textures such as playdough wrapped in plastic. Alternatively, professional leather-lined blindfolds are sold in most sex shops, and are inexpensive.

The person being blindfolded is going to experience more sensory sensitivity in the other areas so even mundane activities can take on a whole new meaning. You could get someone, for instance, to try eating dinner blindfold, or taking a (supervised) bath and let them experience their skin with their super-heightened sense of hearing and touch. In this state you can really appreciate erotic massage, being fed a range of raw fruits or being kissed by someone who alternates between drinking something hot and cold. It's all about surprise and anticipation and you can use this to prolong your foreplay. When you're feeling helpless, the introduction of ice-cube play feels out of this world.

For the ultimate in sensory deprivation, try a floatation tank experience. It's a way of getting the deepest relaxation possible, and one hour of floating is equivalent to four hours of sleep. Search online to find somewhere you and your partner can book adjoining rooms and I'll leave it up to you what happens afterwards…

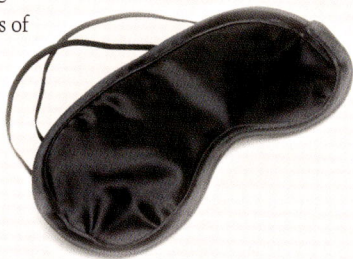

37

Finding it

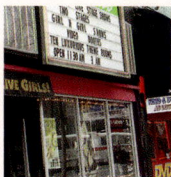

Sometimes staying at home is not where it's at. Try visiting an alternative club, sauna, workshop or sex shop.

Try going to a sauna where you'll actually get to see real women naked: young, old, fat, and everything in between – the experience is normalising. Yep, it's OK not to look like Kate Moss. Even if you feel shy at first (try a woman-only session if you're particularly bothered), you'll wonder what all the fuss was about ten minutes later once you're naked.

Once you've shed some of your inhibitions, you're ready to paint the town red. You could try going to different clubs.

Many straight women feel at home in a gay club where any interaction is free from the 'meat-market' mentality of regular clubs. You might even want to try a fetish club. Normally there is a dress code (leather, latex, uniform) but once you're inside you'll find that there's plenty to watch without having to be a 'player'. You don't have to do anything sexual, but it's a chance to open up and find something new to turn you on – and you'll be telling your friends all about it for weeks afterwards.

If the very thought of going to a fetish club leaves you cold, visit a sex shop. Many are women-friendly, well-lit and offer a discreet, professional service. When I persuaded a friend into one, she was pleasantly surprised. Do anything, but do something!

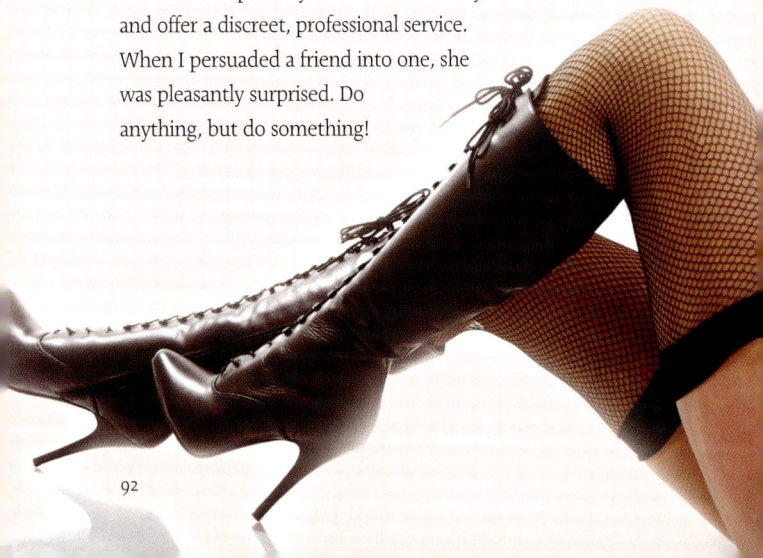

38
Girls on film

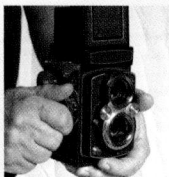

Anything from taking photos to making your own home movie can be an incentive to keep the passion flowing.

Capturing some of your sex life on tape helps to make it seem more real, and a lot of it is going on; video cameras now come in the top twenty list of sex toys.

Perhaps you'll feel more comfortable photographing yourself in private first. This exercise is a great excuse to buy something sexy. You can set up a video camera and leave it running whilst you practice walking, undressing, posing or even masturbating. Play it back to yourself later and note how you moved and how any clothes you wore suited you. You could also use the photo function on your mobile phone to snap all kinds of strange positions down there, or set up a regular camera to go off at timed intervals.

Now you're ready to experiment. Perhaps you're choreographing everything around a narrative – like a sexy nurse and a sick patient. Take the chance to flesh out your fantasies. Later you can analyse your foreplay strategies and put a voice to the images, telling your lover what things turned you on the most. It's a chance to learn something and develop trust, and it might turn you on: it's really the perfect rainy day activity!

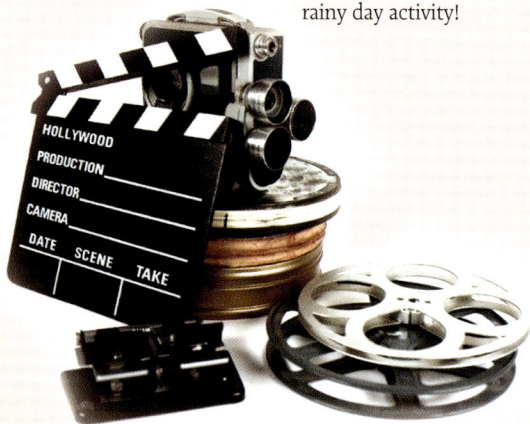

39

Get close

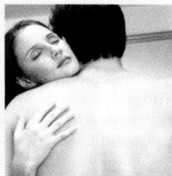

Sometimes touching, cuddling and kissing are more important than intercourse. That's great for cats — here's how to move it from cosy to rosy.

If you both agree that it's time to get back in the driving seat for sex, you need to find some way of jerking you back into action.

Setting aside an afternoon or evening for pleasure is a good start. If you don't feel like sex yet, then mutual masturbation or oral sex is a sexual activity that's just a zone up from the comfort barrier of cuddling. If even this is too much, at least make your kissing more strident; if you've been doing soft, mushy kisses turn these into passionate ones with tongues.

It's easier if the woman initiates a sexual interest. Fondle him suggestively when he's in the shower or make your cuddles go a little more in the direction of the genitals. Better still, try to go out more and arouse his interest in a place where you can't easily cuddle. For example, go out to dinner and whisper sweet nothings in his ear in the restaurant or pass him suggestive notes. Hopefully, it'll make him anticipate something exciting happening later.

To avoid the just-cuddling syndrome, develop a code word or phrase, something you wouldn't normally say – like 'red fizz' – and use this to indicate that you're feeling positively amorous. You could also experiment with a certain type of kiss that signals the same thing; slipping your tongue in his mouth in a smooch lets him know you want it to go further than a cuddle.

40

First time

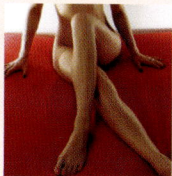

There is lots of evidence showing that delaying sex until you are ready for it makes for more satisfying orgasms.

Virginity is becoming fashionable again. It's OK to delay sex, or not to have sex, but your first experience can affect your sexual development, so look before you leap. The first time you have sex has one of the biggest influences on your sexual future, so if you're going to do it make sure that it's a good experience.

Of course, being a virgin doesn't mean you don't get to have orgasms. On the contrary, you're more likely to masturbate and perfect the art of doing this. If you're able to do this yourself, you're much more likely to have a better sexual frisson with someone else. Debra Boxer wrote an extremely erotic Nerve.com essay, *Innocence in Extremis*, about being a virgin at the age of twenty-eight. Here she describes a particularly satisfying masturbation experience: 'After, my hands shake as if I'd had an infusion of caffeine. I press my hand, palm down, in the vale between my breasts, and it feels as if my heart will burst through my hand.'

Try masturbating at the same time for three consecutive days. How long does it take to get to a state where you can't stop? If you're considering sex with a partner, you'll be able to compare your arousal state, and until you reach that point don't go any further – you're unlikely to orgasm if you do.

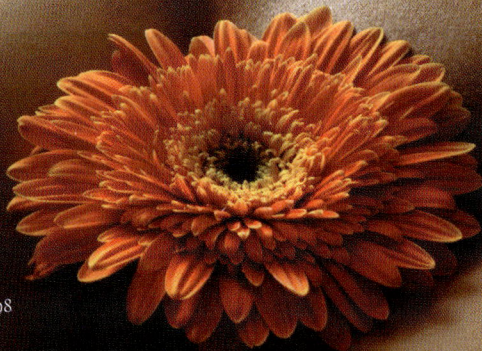

41

The rake

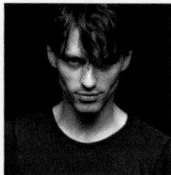

Deep down it's the thrill of no-holds-barred, testosterone-fuelled sex that that attracts us to devil-may-care types. They're assertive, exciting and glamorous — do you want a piece of the action?

If your longing for a bad guy is just a cover for your pent-up desires, it's better for you to play this out yourself rather than waiting passively for someone to do it for you. (Bad boys are notorious, a bit like married men, for promising the world then failing to deliver.) Start by sending out the kind of signals that reflect your real personality. If you want to wear that short skirt, even though it doesn't look 'respectable', just do it. Even if you need to wear something conservative to work, you can wear naughty undies underneath.. Remember you need to unlock your own feelings, with the bad guy as an aide, rather than a bind.

Pay attention to your fantasy life. What really turns you on? And what's stopping you from carrying it out? Don't forget he's the mirror to what you want, not the key to the mysteries of the universe. If you make the focus on you, and why you're attracted to him, it'll allow you to lick all the cream without getting sucked in. Bad boys should be regarded as playthings for a rainy day, and accepted as the risk they are. Enjoy the insights they bring you, but remember they're bound to let you down eventually.

Write down the actual benefits your own bad guy has brought to your sex life. You might be surprised at how little you've experimented so far, so why not come up with your own list? After all, you might as well take full advantage of what's on offer.

42

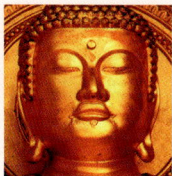

Asian secrets

Steep yourself in the mysterious wonders of Tantric sex and relax into an amazing, pure energy orgasm

Beginning couples can start by bathing together to relax each other, looking deeply into each other's eyes and performing loving rituals like shampooing hair or cleansing. For the next stage move to a sensuous environment, such as a bedroom that has been pre-arranged with candles, incense sticks or flowers. Next use essential oils like sandalwood or bergamot and take it in turns to gently massage each other.

Now you need to practise your breathing to begin the meditation. Sit facing each other and use cushions to get your heads at about the same height. Try to breathe, concentrate on your genitals and expel your breath out in the direction of your vagina. Both of you should be concentrating on doing this, and when you feel it's working look at each other and try to change the flow of the energy. Take the imaginary breath from your genitals and imagine breathing it into your partner's heart.

You can use visualisation techniques, breathing and focus to attain a state of deep relaxation, and then in this state you can begin foreplay and sex. You're aiming to make sexual contact much more than genital stimulation, so try to feel as if you are making love to the whole of your partner's body.

To prolong lovemaking and withhold ejaculation, just before the point of no return flex your PC muscles tight and hold the position. The feeling of needing to orgasm should subside slightly, and then you can resume. Both your and your partner can have a go at this advanced trick. The real deal though is the meditation side: focus that breath!

43

Sex as sport

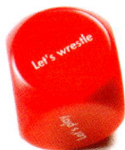

Casual sex can be an emotional minefield so here's how to have the spark without getting burned.

Just thinking about the possibility of casual sex means lots of anticipatory pleasure. The advantage of seeking out a casual partner is that you can discount a lot of the attributes you'd look for in a long-term partner, and can go for attractiveness and sex appeal over a good sense of humour. As long as you tell someone where you're going (should anything occur) and have your got little bag of tricks handy (containing essentials like condoms, clean knickers, make-up, mobile) you're free to take advantage of what's on offer.

Many one-night stands are fuelled by alcohol which is a big passion killer, so don't get too wasted. Ideally, once you're in a suitable location, you should be able to pick up where you left off. Initiate things by kissing and hugging first. Aim to give and receive as much foreplay as possible (crap conquests lead to a rushed orgasm, and its benefits are largely psychological). Talk dirty if it turns you on, and don't be afraid to use any sex toys you have with you, or to experiment with anal sex or different positions. If you've made it clear there's no commitment, don't be afraid to be affectionate, or enjoy multiple orgasms. It's meant to be fun!

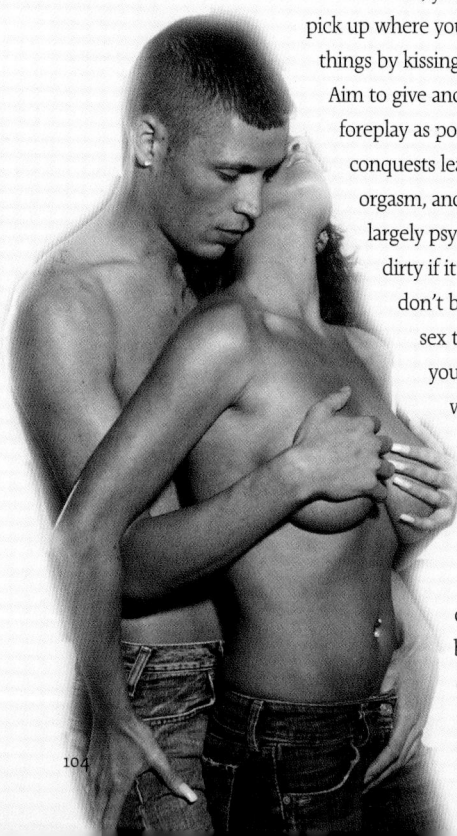

44

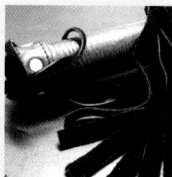

Power to the people

Experimenting with the kinky can lead to mind-opening experiences.

If you're going to try S and M games always agree on everything first and initiate things slowly; it's a bit like foreplay but with more options!

Things to try include tying someone up (bondage), tickling (with hand or feather), stroking, spanking, caning and whipping. If you want to try being submissive without all the fancy gear, you can try meting out 'school' type punishments. Bondage adds an element of fantasy (it's one of the most common ones for both men and women). Be wary about using makeshift household items like silk scarves; they are actually like wire in the wrong hands. Always pad areas that you want to bind first (handcuffs should also be padded). If in doubt, raid the kitchen for cling film and mummify your victim (don't cover the face and don't leave it on for more than an hour, though); you could try a little light spanking over the wrapping.

Adding a little pain to the proceedings is stimulating for some because it releases endorphins – the same feel-good chemicals we get when we exercise. Too much is a turn-off, though, and everyone has a different pain threshold. Always remember to warm up each part of the body first; before moving on to harder strokes, you could start with stroking, move on to tickling and progress to hand spanking then possibly using a different implement. Don't forget that faster strokes feel harder simply because the person experiencing it has less time to catch their breath. So take it slowly and experiment.

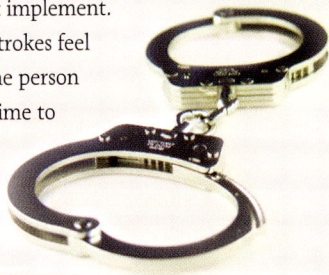

45

Wet scenes

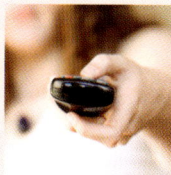

The biggest stumbling block for women is 'getting in the mood' in the first place. A sexy DVD goes a long way into kick-starting something that will inevitably lead to a bit of action.

Some couples use naughty instructional videos, for example Nina Hartley's various guides, Annie Sprinkle's *Fire in the Valley* (1999) and *Becoming Orgasmic* (1994). Director Andrew Blake's porn films also appeal to couples because his work is stylish, the actors attractive and the action women-centred: *see*

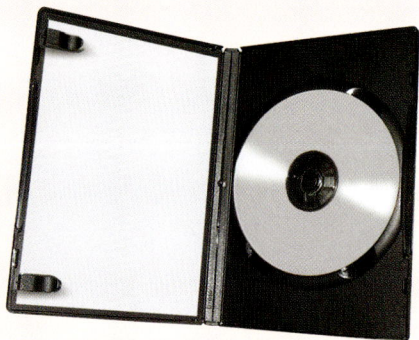

Possessions (1998), *Aria* (2001) and *Hard Edge* (2003). Former porn star Candida Royalle runs Femme which produces soft porn aimed at women; try *Revelations* (1992), *Eyes of Desire* (1998) and *Stud Hunters: A Hard Man is Good to Find* (2003).

The golden age of porn was 1974–1989 where big budgets and good story lines predominated, as in *The Punishment of Anne* (1975), *Sensations* (1975), *The Opening of Misty Beethoven* (1976), *Pretty Peaches* (1978), *Night Dreams* (1983), *Café Flesh* (1983), *Traci I Love You* (1986) and one of my favourites, *Inside Marilyn* (aka *Inside Olinka*, 1985).

In mainstream porn it could be that you don't fancy many of the guys because their main requirement is simply to have a big dick. Try gay porn, where the men will look better (a soft-core example is *Sunshine After the Rain*); it's also a chance to get an insight into another sexual culture.

46

Sheer filth

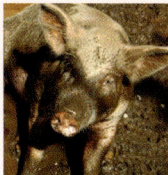

Worrying about how you look, sound or smell can distract you from having that wonderful orgasm. It really is a case of accepting the rough with the smooth.

Having good orgasms means lightening up a bit and becoming more body-tolerant. During sex you have to forget about everything being sterile and prissy clean, even if you've spent hours preparing for the big moment. Our vaginal lips for instance are the sweatiest part of the body and have more sweat glands per inch than our armpits! Dealing with sweat and having to clean up various bodily fluids afterwards is part of the game.

Of course, practising safe sex is the best way to deal with any potential issues. For instance if you want to finger your partner's anus, using a latex glove makes it easy to clean up afterwards without having to scrub your fingernails. Porn actors typically take an enema before any action (although the poo should be out of reach in the colon anyway). We need to become more clued up about safe sex, and to stop worrying about getting the sheets dirty!

Of course, some people like to be dirty. Napoleon forbade his wife to wash for two weeks before he came home from battle; he loved her natural pong! Men are conditioned by porn to believe women love to be ejaculated on – always stipulate what is acceptable. You don't have to do anything extreme, but stop fretting about getting all hot and sweaty.

Practising 'water sports' helps you feel more at ease with your body. Urine is sterile, and if you can let yourself go and actually pee on your partner in the bath or shower (you choose where on his body) you shouldn't have performance anxiety in the throes of orgasm.

47

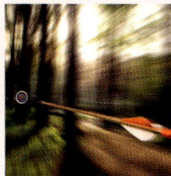

Two easy routes to faster orgasm

Quicker, harder, faster? How to come more easily.

Tweaking your usual lovemaking pattern can improve your sex life with a minimal amount of effort.

Squeezing

When you orgasm, your pubococcygeal (PC) muscles in the vagina contract rapidly. Tighten your PC muscles as he withdraws, and relax them as he enters. It'll take a bit of practice but this is a recommendation from the queen of the female orgasm, Betty Dodson, who through her workshops and books has taught thousands of women how to come, and how to come better. Squeezing will jump-start your own orgasmic contractions.

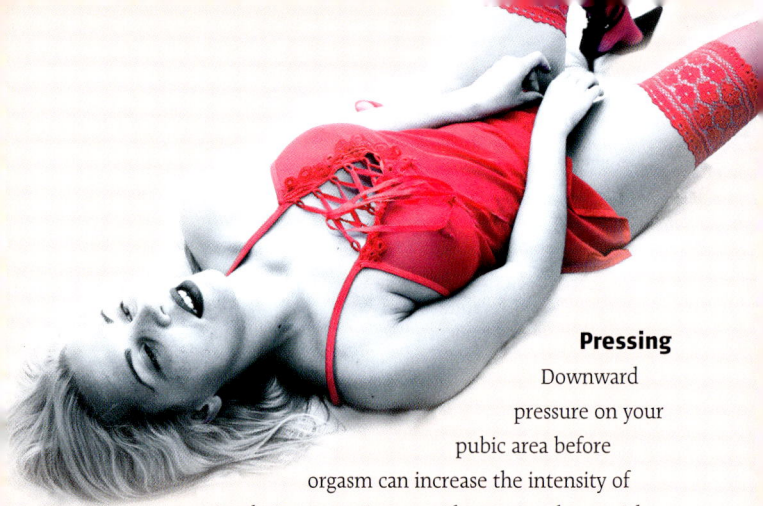

Pressing

Downward pressure on your pubic area before orgasm can increase the intensity of stimulation. Experiment with pressing down with your hand on your stomach just above your pubic bone while masturbating or using a vibrator. Then try this during intercourse. Another technique is to 'bear down'. This is pushing out with your PC muscles, which may help force your G-spot closer to your vaginal opening so it's likelier to get indirect stimulation from his penis.

48

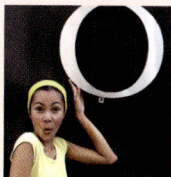

More easy routes to faster orgasm

How to increase your chances of simultaneous orgasm.

Let your partner know how excited you are and encourage the same feedback from him. If you want to minimise prosaic chat, whisper a number to your mate to let him know exactly where on a scale of 1 to 10 you are in terms of getting your rocks off. He can do the same.

Stretching
Stretching your legs flat on the bed and bringing them together while in the missionary position will increase clitoral stimulation. It works even better when you're on top.

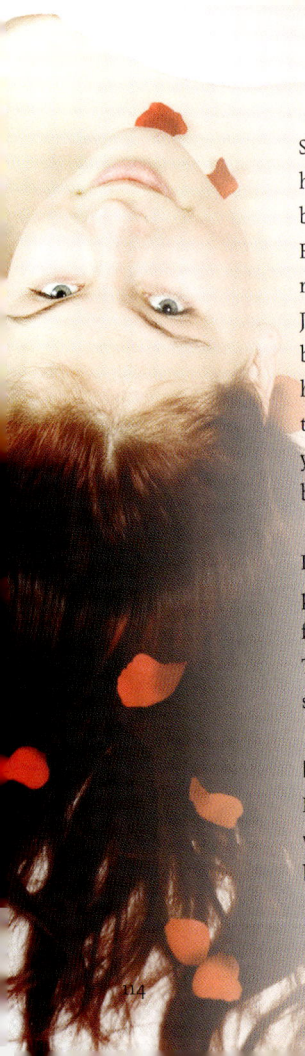

Slide your thighs down so they are over his thighs rather than his hips. Arch your back so you're bending backwards. Forming an arc means you'll be putting maximum pressure on the clitoral area. Just be careful you don't bend his penis back too far – you have all the control here and being a gent he might not want to interrupt your obvious pleasure to tell you that you're in imminent danger of breaking it off.

It's also worth experimenting with other positions where you are on top and your feet are stretched down towards his feet. These tend to increase clitoral stimulation.

Hanging

Hang your head over the edge of the bed when you're having sex. The rush of blood to the brain increases sensations.

49

Handy work 1

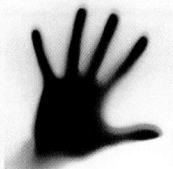

Bringing your partner off with your hand is a staple of a good sex life.

We get into habits with achieving orgasm, just like everything else. We are welded to one way of stimulating ourselves to climax and then (if we're lucky) our partners get proficient at mimicking us and that's the sort of stimulation we get from them. Terrific. No one's knocking that, but ringing the changes and using a different technique can teach you a lot about your sexual response and can result in deeper orgasms. It starts off as a frustrating process – it takes a while to retrain yourself – but rely on the Tantric principle, 'It's the journey not the arrival that's important.' Doing this will make you closer as a couple and it will make you more orgasmic.

Experiment with the following techniques when you're masturbating – once you've got the hang of them, share your new knowledge with your partner. Remember, if you're the one doing the stimulating, don't chop and change between techniques too much in one session, as it's distracting, especially when your partner's approaching orgasm.

Make a fist, place it on the top of the vulva and move it from there. Experiment with position and pressure until you find what works best. Careful, because it's easy to ruin the mood by being too enthusiastic – this one needs lots of communication.

After rubbing the clitoral area with fingers, moving onto a palm provides an intense pressure and an intense orgasm. Using the heel of the palm to grind against the clitoris while the fingers are free to play around with the vagina, perineum and labia gives strong contractions, especially if you press down just above the pubic bone at the same time with your other hand. If you're doing this to your partner, it works well in positions where they are free to grind against the heel of your palm.

50

Handy work 2

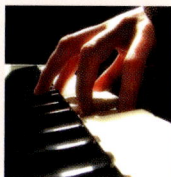

Two more techniques for manual dexterity

The wishbone, sometimes known as 'the V', uses the whole of the clitoris and not just the little nub that we call the clitoris – that's just the bit we see. Spreading outwards and downwards from the clitoris nub, on either side of the vagina and under the skin are the arms of the clitoris. Place your index and middle fingers pointed downwards towards the vagina, one on each side of the labia with the junction of the V on your clitoris nub. Massage the clitoral arms and the clitoris with the V, keeping up constant pressure on all parts of the clitoris. The orgasm from this technique takes time, but that builds tension and gives most women a more diffuse orgasm that's more of a whole body experience. Partners can

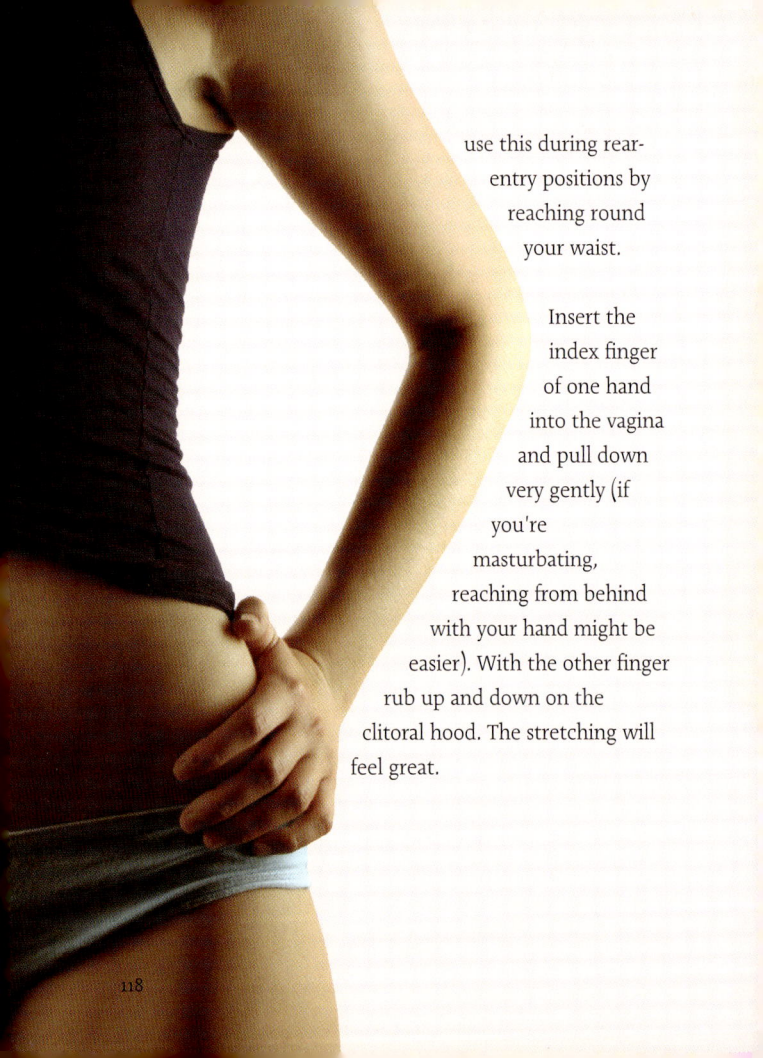

use this during rear-
entry positions by
reaching round
your waist.

Insert the
index finger
of one hand
into the vagina
and pull down
very gently (if
you're
masturbating,
reaching from behind
with your hand might be
easier). With the other finger
rub up and down on the
clitoral hood. The stretching will
feel great.

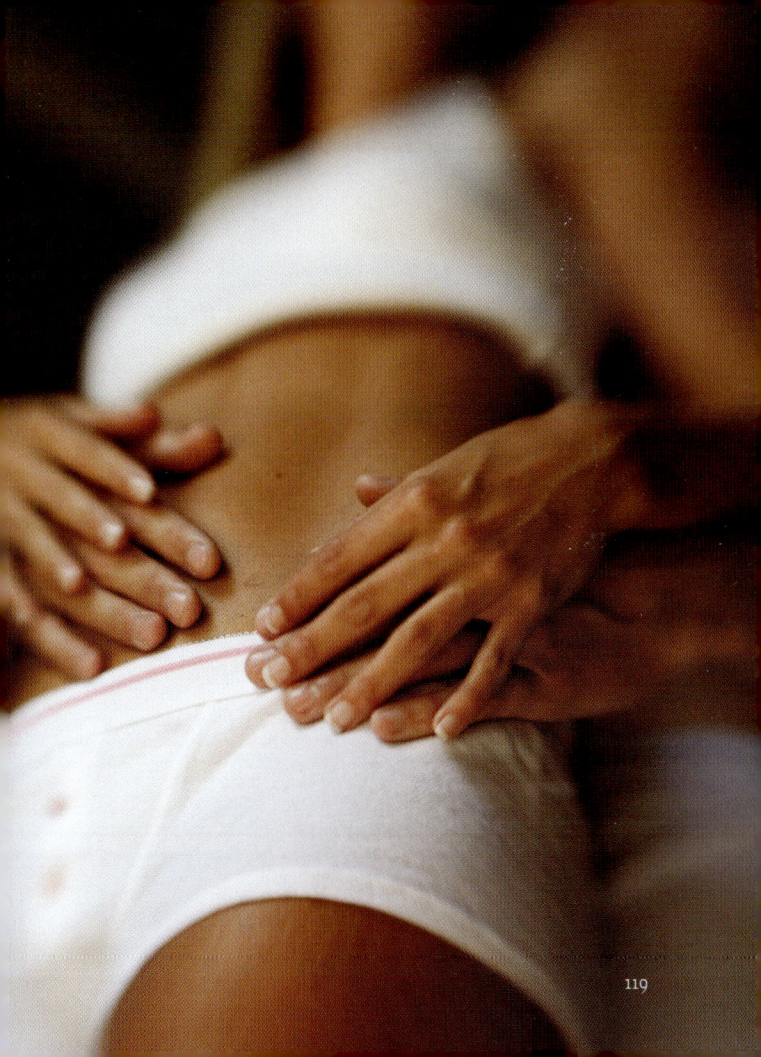

"Women need a reason to have sex, men just need a place"

BILLY CRYSTAL, City Slickers

51

Building bridges

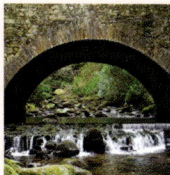

How can a woman come just like a man?

The great majority of women need clitoral stimulation with either hand or vibrator if they're going to come during penetrative sex. Still the ideal persists that we should all be multiorgasmic by penile insertion. Frankly, it's rubbish. The only hope for the vast majority of women is to get used to coming during penile penetration through clitoral stimulation.

However, women and men do persist in feeling that they'd like to come from the same thrusting stimulation. And there is a way to do it: bridging. The bridge manoeuvre means simply using clitoral stimulation to bring the woman to the very edge of coming, then desisting and the woman coming following a few thrusts more from the man. This is a three-step process that anyone can learn, although it takes practice. If you get to step two and come that way, you'll still be in a good place.

Step 1: Adopt the position

Find a position that allows maximum clitoral stimulation. It can be the missionary position or any other as long as your hand stimulates your clitoris. Best is the big mama of quick female orgasm: you straddle your partner, pull aside your labia and lean forward so that your clitoris rubs directly against his pelvic bone or sit upright so that you can masturbate your clitoris while on top of him.

Step 2: Bring your mind into play

You're writhing about, touching yourself. Feel yourself getting closer to orgasm? No? OK, time to bring fantasy into the act. With fantasy, you stop worrying about everything else and concentrate on sex. Concentrate on achieving your orgasm. Shut your eyes. Forget about your bloke if necessary. Don't stop until you come, or if you want to bridge...

Step 3: Bridging

Take yourself to the very edge of orgasm and then stop the clitoral stimulation. Bring yourself off by grinding yourself against his body. This is partly a mental thing. When you believe you're going to come through penetration only, it's more likely that you will.

52

Tongue tricks

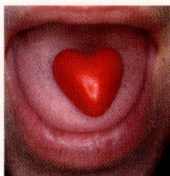

What are the favourite clitoral pleasers?

- Big flat licks using the whole tongue. The wetter the better.
- Flicking up the edges of the labia, eventually centring on the clitoris.
- Licking upwards repeatedly along the furrows from the vagina to the clitoris, gradually pressing harder every time but never quite reaching the clitoris (stimulating the 'arms', you see).
- Licking gently while pressing down just above the mons (the fleshy bit, at present directly above your nose) with the fingers.
- Circle, circle, flick, flick, flick. Circle, circle, flick, flick, flick.
- Very lazy circles around the clitoris, but not touching it. The slower the better at first and then a bit of a build-up can drive you mad with longing.

- Suck the clitoris very gently and flick your tongue over it. Or move the tongue slowly up-down, up-down.
- Make your tongue pointy and insert it into the hole rhythmically. (Author's note: many men overdo this. Remember, the clitoris is the seat of oral sex pleasure. Don't overdo tongue penetration unless specifically asked – assuming that their tongue should mimic their penis is the biggest technical mistake men make.)

Try all of these. And at the end when she's approaching orgasm, he'll probably be doing some version of lapping at your clitoris up and down, firmly and rhythmically in a steady and purposeful manner. You'll be bucking against him now. You might like him to hold onto your buttocks or hands tight as you approach orgasm. It helps you concentrate. Don't change what you're doing at all except perhaps to go a little faster.

Explain to him that the secret to giving great oral sex is to remember that *you* have to be able to concentrate. He needs to help you to stay connected to what's happening to you sexually, but still be able to give over control entirely to him. Once you're approaching orgasm, you don't want to be distracted by him changing what he's doing if he's clearly doing something right.

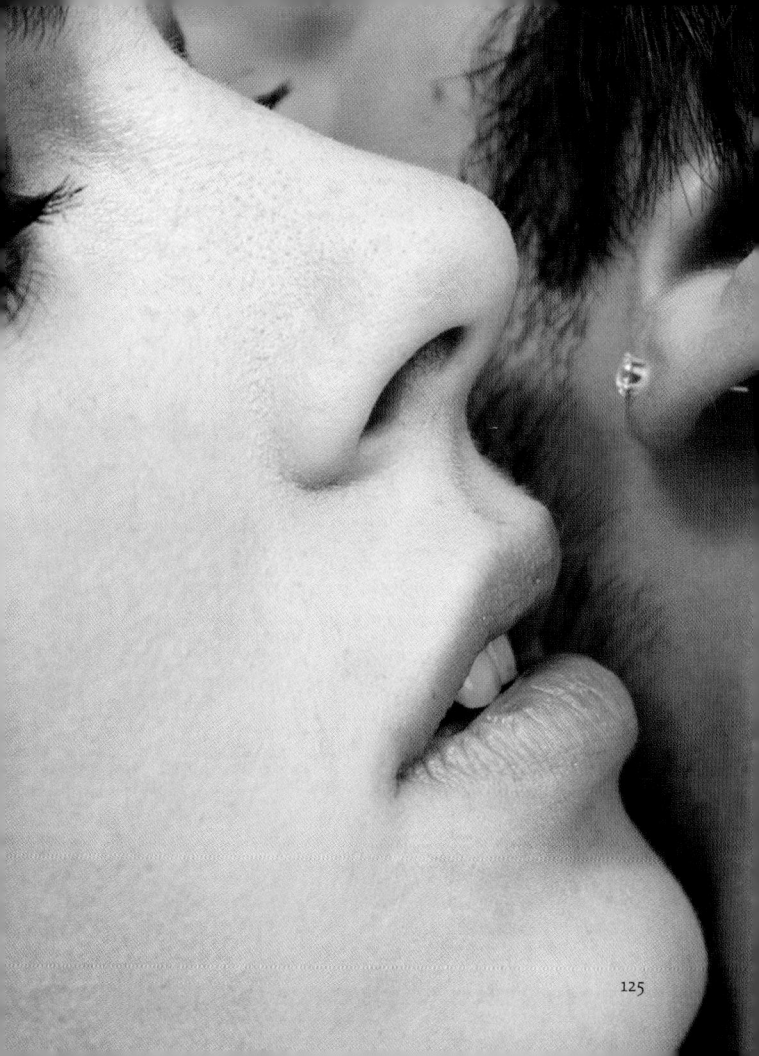

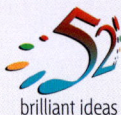

The little book of BIG Os: Brilliant ideas to take you to the limit is published by Infinite Ideas, creators of the acclaimed **52 Brilliant Ideas** series. If you found this book helpful, you may want to take advantage of this special offer exclusive to all readers of *The little book of BIG Os*. Choose any two books from the selection below and you'll get one of them free of charge*. See overleaf for prices and details on how to place your order.

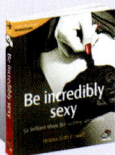

Be incredibly sexy
52 brilliant ideas for
sizzling sensuality

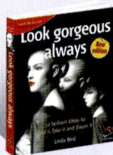

Look gorgeous always
52 brilliant ideas to find it,
fake it and flaunt it

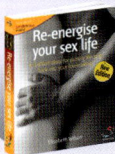

Re-energise your sex life
52 brilliant ideas to put the
zing back into your lovemaking

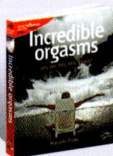

Incredible orgasms
yes, yes, Yes, YES, YESSS!

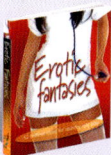

Erotic fantasies
Brilliant ideas for raunchy
role play

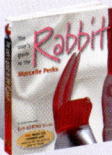

**The user's guide to the
Rabbit**

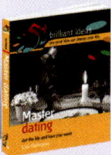

Master dating
Get the life and love
you want

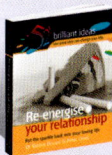

**Re-energise your
relationship**
Put the sparkle back into
your loving life

For more detailed information on these books and others
published by Infinite Ideas please visit www.infideas.com

*Postage at £2.75 per delivery address is additional.

Choose any two titles from below and receive the lowest price one free

Qty	Title	RRP
	Be incredibly sexy	£12.99
	Look gorgeous always	£12.99
	Incredible orgasms	£12.99
	Re-energise your sex life	£12.99
	Erotic fantasies	£6.99
	The user's guide to the Rabbit	£6.99
	Master dating	£12.99
	Re-energise your relationship	£12.99

Subtract lowest priced book if ordering two titles

Add £2.75 postage per delivery address

TOTAL

Name: ....

Delivery address: ....

....

....

E-mail:...........................Tel (in case of problems):..................

By post Fill in all relevant details, cut out or copy this page and send along with a cheque made payable to Infinite Ideas. Send to: *Big Os* BOGOF, Infinite Ideas, 36 St Giles, Oxford OX1 3LD. **Credit card orders over the telephone** Call +44 (0) 1865 514 888. Lines are open 9am to 5pm Monday to Friday. Just mention the promotion code 'LBBOAD07.'

Please note that no payment will be processed until your order has been dispatched. Goods are dispatched through Royal Mail within 14 working days, when in stock. We never forward personal details on to third parties or bombard you with junk mail. This offer is valid for UK and RoI residents only. Any questions or comments please contact us on 01865 514 888 or email info@infideas.com.